CAN'T KEEP SILENT

A Woman's 22-year Journey of
Post-Abortion Healing

Lydia A. Clarke

TATE PUBLISHING, LLC

Scripture quotations marked "KJV" are taken from the *Holy Bible, King James Version,* Cambridge, 1769.

Scripture quotations marked "NIV" are taken from the *Holy Bible, New International Version* ®, Copyright © 1973, 1978, 1984 by International Bible Society. Used by permission of Zondervan Publishing House. All rights reserved.

HE TOUCHED ME. Words and Music by William J. Gaither. Copyright © 1963 William J. Gaither, Inc. All rights controlled by Gaither Copyright Management. Used by permission.

WHITER THAN SNOW. *Words by* James L. Nicholson, in *Joyful Songs No. 4* (Philadelphia, Pennsylvania: Methodist Episcopal Book Room, 1872).

This book is designed to provide accurate and authoritative information with regard to the subject matter covered. This information is given with the understanding that neither the author nor Tate Publishing, LLC is engaged in rendering legal, professional advice. Since the details of your situation are fact dependent, you should additionally seek the services of a competent professional.

ISBN: 1–5988611–4-X

This book is dedicated to hurting women
and men who suffer in silence.

Acknowledgments

It's been a long journey, and I wouldn't have made it without help along the way. Primarily, I give thanks to God, my Father, His precious Son, Jesus, and the Holy Spirit, who is the Spirit of Truth and my Comforter. I also extend sincere and heartfelt thanks to:

My husband and better-than-best friend, Tim, for loving me the way Paul admonished men to love their wives in Ephesians 5. What a special man you are. Thanks for always demonstrating God's unconditional love. This is for life.

My wonderful, individually unique children, Justin, Christen, Kelley, Caleb and Quentin. You are the blessings the Lord promised you'd be. Thanks for your patience and understanding.

My parents, including my stepfather, for your faithful support in all I've aspired to do. Mom, I admire your valor in encouraging me to obey God and complete this book. I know it's difficult, but it truly shows your love for Him and your love for me.

My spiritual father and mother, Dr. Charles and Missionary Donna Hawthorne. I can't even imagine where I'd be without you two. Your supernatural ability to discern, stir and develop latent gifts and callings has propelled me onto a collision course with a destiny and purpose I never imagined existed when I hooked up with your ministry at age 18. Thanks for looking far beyond my faults and into my prophetic future. The Lord has truly given me a pastor and first lady after His own heart.

The Labor of Love Church family, my brothers and sisters. Your support of my family, my ministry, and me has been phenomenal! This book is the fruit of the many seeds you have sown.

Family Life Services. You were there when I needed you most. Susan, you are an instrument of God's peace. Thank you for ministering to me, supporting me and mentoring me for post-abortion ministry.

Lastly, my people, the Jones Family. I love you all. You are the best! Ministry—it's in the bloodline.

Table of Contents

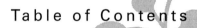

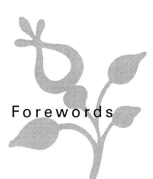

Forewords

I've known Lydia Clarke for well over 20 years. I first met her when I was a Minority Campus Minister at Eastern Michigan University. Four years later, I was privileged to become her pastor. Over the past two decades, I have seen her grow, develop and mature into a woman destined for greatness.

She is a wonderful wife, a devoted mother and an outstanding woman in ministry. I have witnessed her gradual transformation and the difference that Christ has made in her life. She is not the same person she was five, ten, or fifteen years ago. Since her initial salvation, God has delivered, healed and filled her in a way that is nothing short of miraculous. Lydia is a living, breathing, walking, talking testimony of what it means to know the truth and for that truth to set you free.

In this book, she tells her story. And she tells it as only she can. Chapter by chapter, she peels back the layers of her life and lets you see how she was transformed from a victim of abortion to a victor. She gives you a first-hand glimpse of both the tragedy and the triumph.

The good news is that what happened to her can happen to anyone. Anyone can go through something tragic and traumatic and then come out better instead of bitter. This book tells you how.

Pastor C.E. Hawthorne, Senior Pastor
Labor of Love Church
Ann Arbor, Michigan

○○○○○

Many women have fallen prey to this spirit called "abortion," and as a result have literally been held back in their potential to function as successfully as they could in life. There is always that degree of rejection and struggle to get beyond it.

I have heard many women that have experienced abortion say they could hear the cries of their babies in their sleep. They are tormented to the extreme by the enemy of their mind. Many have said that their only hope or recourse was to accept the reality of the situation in its truest form. Only then can they believe to be forgiven and ultimately forgive themselves.

This book will touch the hearts and change the lives of many women. I believe there is a healing balm within the pages of this book. The author has pressed out her inner most being in this writing, and I applaud her transparency and boldness to tell her story.

The daughters of Zion have been represented well. How can women not become whole as a result? This book will blaze the trail for a new generation of writers who also must tell the "Whole Truth," so others can be healed from the residue of pain left behind after an abortion.

This is a heartfelt testimony of God's healing power for all of us who dare to open up the "Pandora's Box" and let the stench come out, so others can also be healed. I trust this will not be the end of the story for Lydia, as there is a need for the masses to hear what is inside of her. I believe a paramount discourse has begun with readers who need to hear a "sistah's" story so they too can find forgiveness, faith, and freedom in order to pursue their purpose and destiny.

Prophetess Veter Nichols
Destiny Ministries
Port Huron, Michigan

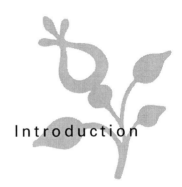

Introduction

I am a Christian, and I am pro-life, but I am *not* pro-life because I am a Christian. Many pro-choice advocates dismiss Christian pro-lifers as religious fanatics who blindly oppose abortion solely based on religion. While I must admit that I am a fanatic, sold out, not to religion, but to Jesus, my beliefs about abortion were not shaped when I became a Christian. No, they formed years before as *I* lay on an abortion clinic's table. My values were certainly strengthened upon learning about the Lord and His ways, but my convictions are unshakable because I experienced the aftermath of abortion firsthand.

The abortion took place in 1976, and if there was a great debate then about when life begins or a woman's right to choose, I was oblivious to it. I lived in a small town, and my family's television received two channels, maybe three if the antenna was positioned just right. The term "abortion" reached my ears only when infrequent rumors of someone having one circulated in my school. Because it was discussed in connection with that same someone being pregnant, I concluded the abortion ended the pregnancy. I attended church regularly because that's what my family did, but the subject of abortion was never addressed there. Without any other influence, my core beliefs concerning abortion stem from my own experience.

Although the procedure itself was traumatic, neither I nor my mother foresaw how that relatively brief moment in my life would emotionally and spiritually handicap me for the next two decades. We couldn't foresee it because we were not forewarned. Generally, prior to a medical procedure, a patient is informed of its associated risks. Armed with this information, the patient then determines whether the procedure is worth the possible negative outcomes. Unfortunately, my mom and I received no information about the potential risk of emotional damage after an abortion. If we had, another decision may have been made. Or, at least it would have been easier to recognize and deal with the root of my suffering.

Instead, the abortion thrust me unarmed onto the front lines of guerilla warfare. My peace, my joy, my self-worth (the little I had), and my womanhood were all being ravaged by an enemy I could not see

- an enemy kept hidden behind the deceptive guises of "a solution to problem," "a woman's right," "legal means safe," "it's nobody's business," or "when it's over, it's over."

The Mandate

As the light of truth exposed my dark enemy, and God's healing balm of love, forgiveness and mercy mended my festering wounds, I emerged from two decades of bondage with a mandate. This mandate demands I speak out.

Psalms 30:11–12 says:

> *Thou has turned for me my mourning into dancing: thou hast put off my sackcloth and girded me with gladness; to the end that my glory may sing praise to thee, and **not be silent**. O Lord my God, I will give thanks unto thee forever. (KJV)*

In healing me from the effects of my abortion, God turned my weeping into joy; He turned my mourning, my grief, into dancing. Why? Just so I could shout, "Yay, I'm healed!"? Absolutely not. This issue is much larger than just me.

There are many post-abortive women who are suffering alone because of shame. They believe they have committed the unpardonable sin, and thus are unwilling to seek help. There are also those who are suffering emotionally, but, as was the case with me, do not connect the abortion to their pain due to the deceptive manner in which abortion is presented. Then there are those who have been emotionally damaged by abortion, but are unaware of the damage; they espouse the belief, "This is just how I am." It's for all these women my heart must sing His praise and not keep silent. My mandate is primarily for them.

Second Corinthians 1:3–4 says:

Blessed be God, even the Father of our Lord Jesus Christ, the Father of mercies, and the God of all comfort; who comforteth us in all our tribulation, that we may be able to comfort them which are in any trouble, by the comfort wherewith we ourselves are comforted of God. (KJV)

In my trouble, the God of all comfort comforted me. Now I must comfort those who are in trouble with the same comfort I received from Him. My passionate desire is that no woman suffers like I did, for as long as I did; thus, I can't keep silent.

In verbally sharing my testimony, I have witnessed its tremendous impact on both men and women alike. In this book, though, I bare the experience with unprecedented depth. This intensely emotional and spiritual account doesn't just present facts about post-abortion trauma and healing. It allows you, the reader, to feel what I felt and experience what I experienced. This in turn enables you to connect with the truths shared on a deeper, personal level - not just intellectually. As a result, I believe post-abortive women will undoubtedly recognize themselves in some aspect of this experience, and connect with the aftermath of their own abortions.

I'll always remember the hand water pump in my grandmother's front yard. The water which flowed from it was cold and delicious, and I and my cousins loved it. However, pumping the handle alone could not access this precious water. In order for the water to flow *out,* water had to be poured *into* the pump, breaking the vacuum that held it underground. God uses this testimony as water poured into the pump of other post-abortive women's hearts, breaking the vacuum of denial, shame and loneliness, allowing their emotional pain to flow, so He can heal them. This book is not just a story or another autobiography; it is a catalyst for healing.

Exposing myself in this manner is no easy task. However, I must allow the Father to use me as a voice to proclaim the truth about the consequences of abortion. Women are fighting for the right to choose, but a sound choice cannot be made based on partial facts. Full counsel precipitates good choices. Unfortunately, what's prevalent in the media concerning abortion is only part of the story. This book will reveal the other side of this horrific choice that not only takes the life of a baby, but cripples a woman's soul. As the truth is revealed, the Lord can set women free from the prison in which the lies of abortion have locked them. John 8:32 says, "And ye shall know the truth, and the truth shall make you free." (KJV)

The Lord wants to set you free through the truth. To accomplish this deliverance, however, all defense mechanisms must be disengaged, and your heart opened. My story is by no means unique, so if you courageously allow your guards to drop and permit Him to connect your dots, you may see a picture of your situation you've never seen before. It may be painful or ugly, but I'm a witness that the picture is not the end. Just remember, if God reveals it, He will assuredly heal it.

Let the truth make you free.

chapter 1

My Moment of Truth

The Set-up

It was a cold December night when I received an unexpected visit from the twins. Lord knows I had missed them. Their visits had been growing more infrequent. On those rare occasions when they were able to slip in, the demands of my seemingly never-ending responsibilities cut our visits short.

Although I don't dwell on it, I do fondly remember the days when the twins were more than just visitors; they were residents. We lived happily together throughout my singlehood and the early days of my marriage. I had always known that my dream of a large family posed the risk that my cherished twins would be sacrificed to the back burner; but it was a risk I was willing to take and a sacrifice I was willing to make. Still, in their absence, the twins were greatly missed.

I assumed that my husband was responsible for this particular visit because he had spontaneously rounded up our oldest three children, ages 12, 11, and 5, and taken them on an outing. It seemed that the twins only stopped by when my ever active, fun-loving, still-can't-use-their-inside-voices children were either asleep or out of the house. For that reason, I assumed that my husband must have taken the children out because he knew that I really needed a visit from the twins.

The cherished twosome, Peace and Quiet, arrived as soon as the door had closed behind my departing family. While my one-year-old son slept soundly on my lap, I relaxed in their company with my feet elevated in our worn, but comfortable brown recliner. Only the light from the television illuminated the room.

It would not be long before I discovered my husband was not the mastermind behind this precious, unexpected moment of tranquility. No, my family's departure, my busy toddler's nap, the stillness of the house, and my "chair potato" position in front of the television all provided the setting for a drama - a drama written, produced and directed by Someone larger than either my husband or me. This unseen Someone sat in His director's chair, behind the scenes, clapping His hands and commanding, "Places everyone! Quiet on the set!"

With everyone now unwittingly in his or her designated place, the show was about to begin. Little did I know that I was the main character in this invisible script, and that this particular scene was setting me up for what would go down in my personal history as the "moment of truth."

The Moment

For about an hour, I sat in the chair, drifting in and out of sleep while the television watched. Right on cue, as the Director would have it, I drifted back into consciousness just in time to vaguely hear a television commercial for an upcoming movie. Hearing its title, "Fifteen and Pregnant," pulled me further out of my sleepy stupor.

I remembered this movie from a couple of years before, but I had never gotten around to watching it. The preview showed scenes of a fifteen-year-old girl finding out that she was pregnant, followed by the understandably dismayed reaction of her parents. Those scenes propelled me backwards in time, back almost twenty-two years, back to the time when I, too, was fifteen and pregnant. The disappointment and sadness on my parents' faces flashed through my mind, and I completely related to the characters in the movie.

As the commercial continued, the movie's plot took an unexpected turn. I watched as the mother and daughter shopped for baby clothes together, smiling and laughing all the while. Lastly, the preview showed scenes of the fifteen-year-old birthing the baby and suggested images of everyone living happily ever after.

That is where my story and the movie's storyline parted company, and I couldn't relate anymore. I muttered to myself, "That didn't happen to me."

After the last mumbled word left my lips, the Holy Spirit ever-so-gently spoke His scripted pivotal one-line in this unfolding drama. He said, "That's how you were violated."

The calm tone of His voice and the brevity of His one-liner belied the extreme force it carried. This simple sentence morphed into a powerful missile guided toward one target, and one alone - the enormous weight that had lodged in my chest many years before.

In an instant, it hit and detonated. Tears began rolling down my cheeks, and whatever had settled in my chest began a slow ascent up toward my mouth; it was on its way out. It felt so large and overwhelming that I began to panic. The impact of what the Lord had said to me occurred so suddenly that my mind was trying desperately to catch up with what was taking place in my soul.

Ordinarily, I yield to the Lord's dealings with me, and I definitely knew He was working, but I was home alone with my baby, and I sensed that what-ever was on its way out was too big for me to handle on my own. Consequently, I sucked in a huge breath of air, swallowed hard, silently convinced myself, "You can't do this now," and suppressed it. I would have to deal with it later. When later was, I did not know, but I did know that my "moment of truth" had finally come.

Looking Back

For years, I had known that something was not quite right with me. There was some unseen defect that kept me from being whole. Though I could not define it, I also could not ignore it. It felt like a weight bearing down on my chest.

Although my husband and I had been married for fourteen years, it was only in recent years that I would occasionally feel uncomfortable with his close presence. At times, when he would stand very close to me, I would say, "You're violating my space." I'd say it jokingly, but somewhere deep beneath the surface I feared I meant it. It hadn't happened often, but these occasions had increased as my moment of truth approached.

God had used me for many years to minister to hurting women. In ministering to those who had been abused, I always recognized some of their pain in me. Naturally, I began to wonder if I had been sexually abused. In trying to find an answer, I read books about inner healing and the healing of memories and considered the possibility that I had blocked out a traumatic experience. I also questioned my mother and oldest sister about it, but neither was aware of any kind of abuse occurring in my past. I struggled trying to remember, praying often, asking the Lord to show me what had happened to give me this sense of injury within.

One Sunday, at my church, I stood at the altar for prayer for this issue. The woman of God ministering to me spoke this prophetic word: "God wants you to know that He will show you, but He will do it when you are ready; so don't worry about it, and don't force it." At that point, I let it go, confident that the Lord knew better than I when I could handle the answer I'd been seeking. I never imagined that He would use a television commercial as a catalyst for this long-awaited revelation.

The truth was that I *had* been violated. However, it was not the kind of violation I'd always suspected. Unlike the pregnant fifteen-year-old in the movie, my pregnancy at fifteen had been terminated by abortion. The Lord had finally revealed to me that this was the source of my sense of violation. I would have never linked the emotional suffering of the past twenty-two years to the abortion. It took the Holy Spirit, who is the Spirit of Truth, to expose that connection. Even further, I did not recognize that abortion was a form of violation.

The Moment of Truth Continues

After I subdued the feelings of panic and was able to process what had just happened, I realized the heaviness rising in my chest was the conglomeration of what I had either suppressed or didn't know existed as a result of the abortion. It was a volcano on the verge of erupting.

I could not conceive in my mind how God was going to heal and deliver me of what I felt in that moment. I did not know where to go, or who to turn to for help. Nevertheless, I was confident that since God revealed it, He would heal it. After all, He is the God that does all things well.

chapter 2

Looking for Love and Acceptance

While ministering to various audiences on the topic of sex or other related issues, I sometimes reveal the age at which I had my first sexual encounter. It never fails that afterward, someone will ask, "What made you have sex at such a young age?" I had to ask myself the same question after looking through adult eyes at children who were the same age as me when I became sexually active. The answer that materialized looked like this . . .

We all have an innate need to be loved, whether we want to admit it or not. What many don't realize is that this need was placed in us by God. I John 4:18 says, " . . . God is love" *(KJV)*. God does not just love us (love as a verb), but He *is* love

(love as a noun). Our need for love is designed to lead us on a quest for love that finds its fulfillment in God Himself.

Unfortunately, our journey is filled with imposters who profess they possess the love for which we long and detours which seemingly lead us away from God, heightening our craving, not just for love, but acceptance, also.

At fifteen, I knew there was a risk of getting pregnant when having sex, especially unprotected sex, but I didn't think it would happen to me. Actually, I believe I just didn't care. I don't mean I *wanted* to get pregnant. It's just that somehow, I had developed the misconception that sex equaled love, and the risk of pregnancy obviously did not outweigh *my* overwhelming need to feel loved and accepted.

I longed for someone to love me, and accept me just as I was. I wanted someone to accept, what I read someone describe as, my "unchangeables." It is one thing to be rejected for things you can change (your attitude, weight, clothing style, for example), but it is quite another to be rejected for things you cannot change and over which you have no control. There are quite a few items on the list of "unchangeables," but the ones for which I received the most rejection were my parents, my heritage, and my physical features.

My quest for the love of God that would ultimately satisfy the longing in my soul took a major detour early in life leaving me feeling rejected and unlovable.

The Detours

As I sat at my desk working on my morning math lesson in my south side Chicago second grade classroom, my stomach felt as if it were turning flips. Every now and then I would glance at the clock, and with every glance lunchtime drew a little closer. It was difficult to concentrate on the addition and subtraction problems, and with my struggle with subtraction, I really needed to focus.

Were the other kids in my class nervous about the "Father Lunch?" I looked around the room, and they appeared calm as they worked on their assignments. I didn't detect any tension or nervousness. Boy, was I jealous. They were probably looking forward to their fathers coming for lunch. Eating at their desks in the classroom, rather than in the cafeteria, probably added to the excitement.

I, too, was looking forward to sharing lunch with my dad, especially since it was rare to see him at school events during the day because he worked hard running his plastic covers business. After leaving for school in the mornings, I generally did not see him again until late in the evening when he returned home after his long commute on Chicago's congested freeways. Today, he was leaving his business, braving the freeways and coming to my school in the middle of the day just to sit and eat lunch with me, and I was honored. It would have been better, though, if we could have enjoyed our special moment alone. The fear of what my friends and their parents would think or say when they saw my dad put a damper on the excitement and filled me with anxiety.

It was my third year at this predominantly black elementary school, so it is highly likely that in the past two years, my dad had visited the school for some other special program. But today would be different. He would not be just another parent in a crowd of parents. He would be sitting with me at my desk in full view of the entire class. Maybe my classmates knew, maybe they did not, but whenever he arrived and sat down at my desk, they all would know for sure that my father was white.

My mother was black, and she assured me that I, too, was black because I had the infamous "one drop of black blood." Consequently, there was no question in my mind that my classmates also knew I was black. It did not matter that my skin complexion was extremely light, and my hair seemed to be much longer and a little straighter than the other black girls. I was just as black as any other black person except I was the only black person I had seen with a white daddy. This made me different, and I did not want to be different.

Being different was akin to wearing a huge sign on my chest saying, "Please make fun of me." Although I was only in second grade, I had already grown weary of comments, jokes and discussions about me and my dad.

In the first grade, while standing in the hall awaiting entrance to our classroom, my classmates decided to settle once and for all the question that apparently had been nagging them for quite some time: "Is Lydia really pretty?" Why this was important enough to spark a class-wide debate escaped me, but I listened intently, wondering myself what the outcome would be. Am I pretty or am I not? Some argued, "Of course, she *is* pretty," while others rebutted, "No she *isn't*." As the door to the classroom opened, indicating it was time to bring the discussion to a close, one boy wrapped it up by concluding, "People who look pretty like her are really ugly, so she's really ugly." It was settled. I was really ugly. I think.

I am fortunate to have a great extended family. My mother has seven sisters and three brothers, who produced countless playmates for me in the form of cousins. My dad's family had little contact with us, but that was of no consequence to me because there was no shortage of loving relatives in my mom's huge, tight-knit family. I often thank God for blessing me with such a wonderful family. They are a fun-loving crew; however, when I was young, part of the fun included making jokes about my dad.

I lived with my parents, two sisters and two brothers in the upper flat of a two-story building. One Christmas or Thanksgiving, our entire family -

grandparents, aunts, uncles, cousins - were gathered in our flat for dinner. We sat at a long table that stretched the entire length of our living room and was filled with all kinds of tasty fare that my mother, grandmother and aunts had prepared. I sat next to one of my cousins with whom I was very close. We were chatting away as little girls do, when my ears picked up a conversation among the adults. I stopped talking and listened as my aunts and uncles made "white man" jokes about my dad. I stared at him in disbelief as he laughed along with them. Nothing they said struck me as funny, so I did not understand why he was laughing. I perceived their jokes as an attack against my father, and because he was the only white person in the room, I felt my large family unfairly outnumbered him. Out of hurt and disappointment, I looked at my cousin and said, "I hate them."

I remained angry throughout the rest of the holiday, but there was no way I could hold a grudge against this special group of folks whom I adored. Eventually, I continued my love relationship with them, but the wound remained.

As I grew older, I came to understand that my family cracked jokes about everyone, and of course, I had my turn at being teased for my thin lips, light-colored skin, thin nose and flat butt. Their philosophy was, "It is tough out there in the real world. We have to toughen you up, so when you get out there, you will be able to take it." I am proud to say my family's overall training and influence, without a doubt, contributed to my development into the strong, well-rounded, take-care-of-business woman I am today. However, their playful jesting with my father and about my physical features, along with periodic scenes like my first-grade experience contributed to my ever-growing insecurity regarding my unchangeables.

This spurred the anxiety about the "Father Lunch." My dad finally appeared in the doorway of the classroom, and a huge smile lit up his face when he spotted me sitting at my desk. He was in his late fifties. His mostly gray, balding hair was cut short and combed straight back, and he sported his usual white short-sleeved shirt (with its pocket filled with pens), and a striped tie. I smiled back and waved my arm, motioning for him to come on over. He sat down in the little chair at my little desk, and I pulled out the sack lunch my mom had prepared for us. Some of my classmates stared, but as we ate our sandwiches and talked, my anxiety dissipated and no one else mattered. He was my dad, and I loved him. The truth was out, but luckily, no one said anything about him.

The Move

Every other weekend, my family packed up the car and drove to my grandparents' home in Michigan. On one visit, my dad ventured across the street to the neighbors' home. The next thing we knew, he had bought their house. We were going to move to Michigan and live right across the street from my grandparents!

Living close to Grandma and Granddad was a dream come true, but the nightmare involved leaving Chicago and our two-and-a-half bedroom flat that served as the setting for my fondest childhood memories. In addition, our new Michigan home was in the middle of nowhere, and we had to drive at least five miles just to go to a store. In Chicago, I had the freedom of walking right around the corner to Mr. Boone's store where I could buy a bag-load of penny-candy and gum, or get a tasty, refreshing snow cone in the summer or one of those huge dill pickles which I would pierce with a peppermint stick straw and suck out the juice. I could ride my bike to the five and ten cents store on Cottage Grove and buy toys, gifts, and of course, more candy. I loved riding the bus and the el (elevated train) around the city with my mom or older sister. In the alley behind our building, I and scores of other kids on the block would play all kinds of games, including my favorite, double-dutch. My heart ached at the thought of losing all this, not to mention having to start a new school and make new friends. Nevertheless, in the summer of 1970, we moved to Michigan.

The New School

My first day at my new school was also my first day of fourth grade. I made new friends quickly, and without any effort at all, I also made enemies. By now, I had grown fairly accustomed to the comments about being "mixed" racially, but these comments were generally made without malice. The kids at my new school, however, were antagonistic and hateful towards me. Girls I barely knew would sneer at me or try to instigate fights with me. I did not understand why I drew out the worst in some people, but I figured it probably had something to do with my light complexion, and what they - and I reiterate, they - described as "good," long hair.

Not only was my dad white, but he was a Jew who immigrated to this country from Poland. I think my previous classmates were unaware of this "twist" in my bi-racial heritage, although my last name, Blumenkrantz, should have been a big clue. My dad told me our surname was German and meant "a wreath of flowers." I was proud of my name and the fact that I could spell it before kindergarten. I was also very pleased that I could legibly write this 12-letter name in the smallest spaces.

In Chicago, kids did not make a big deal out of my name, but in this small, rural, predominantly black community, its uniqueness in pronunciation, spelling (the "z" at the end really topped it off), and sheer length prompted the widespread question, "Where did you get a name like that?" I naively, but proudly, gave the answer. Bad idea.

As I got older and progressed through junior high, my heritage and name became a vicious weapon in the hands of male and female alike who teased me and called me names like, "Jew Jew," "Oreo," and "Half-Breed." I was addressed by demeaning forms of my last name, including "Blumendrawers." Of course today, most of those who teased me would probably say they were just joking as children do. While it is true that children, as well adults, tease and crack jokes, that sort of bantering chipped away at my already weakening self-esteem.

Girls made a point of reminding me that I was not as pretty as I thought (as if I ever thought that), and they constantly threatened me with physical harm just because I brushed back my hair from my face or looked at myself in a mirror. "Look at her. She thinks she's so cute," they would say, even though they spent a lot more time primping their hair and faces.

In addition to my father being a white Jew, he was 25 years older than my mother and most of my peers' parents, as well. He had also suffered a series of strokes that left him partially paralyzed on his right side, so he dragged his leg when he walked. This, too, prompted jokes and snide remarks.

Rejection Sets In

From all I had experienced, I concluded in my child-like understanding that there was something wrong with me and self-hatred, especially of the white part of me, grew. Not only that, but even though I loved my father with all my heart, as I got older and the persecution increased, it became more and more difficult to express that love because I blamed him for my hardships. If he had just been black, my life would have been easier. I know this sounds irrational because I'm sure if I had been brought up among whites, I would've been persecuted for being black. However, as a child, this was my perception, and it resulted in an even deeper longing to be loved and accepted. Unfortunately, like countless others throughout the ages, I thought that an intimate relationship with someone would satisfy that need.

My First "Love"

My boyfriend and I started "going together" when I was thirteen years old. I believed I was in love with him, and he was in love with me.

Today, I have had three children reach the age of 13, and after observing their immaturity both emotionally and physically at that age, I cannot believe I thought I knew what love was about. I cannot fathom why I thought I was mature enough to have sex. What was I thinking? Well, I suppose I wasn't thinking. I just wanted to be loved.

We spent as much time together at school as we could. When I was about fourteen, my parents allowed him to visit me at home. We would talk for hours about any and everything, listen to music and dance.

I never told my parents about my troubles at

school, so they never had the opportunity to help or comfort me. In fact, the more trouble my peers gave me, the bigger the gulf grew between me and my dad. We had a love-hate relationship. I loved him very much and he was a wonderful father to me, but I hated him because, again, it was his fault people wanted to beat me up. So the only comfort I found was with my boyfriend. Being with him helped ease the pain of rejection and somewhat filled my need for love. But, of course, it wasn't enough. Anything outside of God will never be enough. I hungered for more, and I believed I knew how to get it. I gave him my virginity.

One day in January, 1976, my mom called when I returned home from school and told me my father was in intensive care at the hospital. He had suffered with sickness for most of my life, which undoubtedly contributed to the insecurity with which I struggled because I never knew if he would live or die after one of his strokes or heart attacks. I do not recall if he had a stroke or heart attack this time, but here we were again - Is he going to live or die? I was afraid. I did not want him to die. So I followed my usual course of action when things went awry; I sought love and comfort through intimacy with my boyfriend.

The Split-Second Decision

He told me to get up; he was about to climax. I heard him. I understood what he said, but I hesitated. Why did I hesitate? Through the years since then, I have asked myself that question many times. As a matter of fact, my boyfriend asked me that question. I didn't know then, and I don't know now. Sometimes my children do crazy things, and when I ask them why, they simply respond, "I don't know." I can relate. That split-second decision changed my life forever.

chapter 3

Finding Guilt and Shame

Not yet aware that my split-second decision had set in motion a flurry of activity within my body, my life as a high school freshman continued as it had before. My dad was recovering well at home, and schoolwork kept me busy.

I suspected my period might be late. I had never done a good job keeping track of its due date, but I felt like it should have come already. The familiar, but dreaded PMS symptoms were present and accounted for, but there was no blood. Some days I was certain it had started, so I would hurry to the bathroom to secure protection, only to discover it really had not begun. My body seemed to be playing tricks on me. As days passed with no period, anxiety began to mount as I considered, but continually denied, the possible reason for the delay in my cycle.

I began to get very tired. As soon as I'd return home from school, the sofa on our porch drew me like a magnet to its soft cushions, where I would collapse and immediately fall sound asleep. At times, while in school, extreme sleepiness would overtake me to the point where my neck seemed to be screaming out, "I can't hold up this head any longer!" I reasoned that it wouldn't hurt to lay my head down on the desk just for a minute. You know, to give my neck some relief. Before I realized I had fallen asleep, someone would be shaking me out of unconsciousness, informing me the bell had rung, and it was time to go to the next class.

My young nephew and niece's usual resting place on my lap was temporarily shut down due to the pain shooting through my breasts whenever they laid their heads on my chest. Even laying on my stomach became an impossible feat because of the tenderness of my breasts. I had not been educated in the symptoms of pregnancy, but as these strange changes in my body and the absence of my period continued, I deduced I was probably pregnant.

Now what? Who would I tell? How would I get help? I desperately went over and over it in my mind. If I were really pregnant, my parents would be disappointed and hurt, so I certainly could not tell them. I was an A-student, and they expected great things from me. The last thing I wanted to do was hurt my parents.

Countless women find themselves pregnant in less-than-perfect circumstances. Mine was being a fifteen-year-old whose greatest need was to be loved and accepted. Now I was anticipating receiving just the opposite - massive rejection from parents, relatives, friends, teachers - everybody I really cared about. I'm not referring to the kind of rejection where people push you out of their lives, but the kind that comes from being looked upon as a disgrace and a failure. I was terrified.

One day, during lunch period at school, I revealed my suspected pregnancy to my boyfriend. We had a routine of eating lunch together, then going to a little nook in the school building's hallway where we would spend the rest of the period talking and kissing. When I broke the news to him in our special place, he was very calm and comforting. I, on the other hand, was an emotional wreck. I had been pushed over the top by the combination of the impending upheaval in my life, finally telling someone my secret, and what I now understand as the major hormonal changes attributed to pregnancy.

Before I could get myself together, the bell rang ending lunch. Students filled the hallway, and my hysteria was apparent to all who glanced my way. Two girls, who later became my best friends, approached me and asked what was wrong. I couldn't tell them. I really wanted to tell them because I knew they were asking out of sincere concern, but I was too ashamed. A few moments later, another girl, who I knew meant me no good, asked me the same question, and I told her. To this day, I still do not know what motivated me to tell her. This was another bad decision on my part. Needless to say, the word of my suspected pregnancy spread like wildfire, and eventually reached my home.

Confrontation with My Mother

I remember so clearly the night when my mom called me into the kitchen to talk with me. She told me she had heard rumors that I might be pregnant, and asked if it was true. Butterflies fluttered in my stomach, and my eyes stung as tears began to form. God only knows when or if I would have ever voluntarily shared this information with her. Nevertheless, what I had dreaded for weeks was now upon me. She knew. I gathered all the courage I could, looked at her face and said, "Yes." This happened almost thirty years ago, so I cannot remember all the words that were spoken in this difficult confrontation, but the hurt and disappointment contorting my mother's face is forever engrained in my memory. I had done what I never wanted to do - let her down. The guilt was almost unbearable for me, but I knew there was more to come. She had to tell my father.

The next morning, I lay in bed dreading what I would face when I entered the kitchen where my mom and dad usually sat drinking their morning coffee. I figured my mother had probably told my dad sometime during the night, and in my mind I tried to picture how he would look at me. Would it be a look of disappointment, anger, or sadness? I desperately wanted to escape; just seep into a wall and disappear. But I knew I had to face him.

The Numbing Begins

When a person experiences a debilitating pain like a headache, toothache or muscle ache, he or she will usually take medication to numb the ache, enabling them to function at a somewhat normal capacity. In order for me to get out of bed and face my mother and father's pained reactions to my pregnancy that morning, I had to numb myself emotionally. There was no other way. This was the beginning of the self-anesthetization process that continued over the next few weeks, enabling me to function despite the shame, guilt and loneliness. At the time, I had no idea what I was doing - this realization came much later. I just did what was necessary to face another day.

As I walked into the kitchen, I could see my father's back and mother's face. I looked at my mom and saw her swollen eyes; I knew she had been crying. Crying is not something my mom did often, but from the looks of her eyes, she had cried a lot through the night. She had cried because of me. More guilt, more pain, so more numbing. My dad turned around and looked at me. There was no single emotion I saw in his face, but the longer he stared, the more ashamed I felt.

I do not recall what happened after that; I do not know what my dad said to me. All I know is my parents were hurt and disappointed, and it was not the result of anything my four siblings had done; it was because of me. More anesthetic, please.

chapter 4

The Decision

While writing this book, the Lord awakened me early one morning and began to speak to me about this chapter. He told me that I could not give a full, accurate account of the decision-making process because the decision, for the most part, was my mom's. He told me to ask her to write about what influenced her in the decision to abort. I knew this prompting was from the Holy Spirit because I would have never thought to ask this of my mother. Never. But He was right. She could best describe what led her to make this decision. Not only that, but when I share my testimony, people only hear my side. Upon hearing that it was my mother's decision, without hearing her side, they draw inaccurate conclusions about her. It is only fair to document the struggle she faced in making this decision. Here are her words.

ooooo

These words from an old familiar hymn "shackled with a heavy burden, 'neath a load of guilt and shame," come to mind as I reflect on my mental state those many years ago that my daughter wants me to remember and put to paper.

Shackled with the burden of making a decision that would affect my innocent, quiet, beautiful fifteen-year-old daughter was a great weight on my soul. Shackled with guilt that I had been a less-than-diligent watchman and shame that neither her father, nor I, nor any member of our closely knit family had been alert enough to see and meet her need for more love, comfort, and consolation. Her father was, at the time, having a difficult time recuperating from a serious operation, and we were totally caught up in his struggle.

I can't remember to this day how I found out she was pregnant. All I remember is crying out in my spirit "Lord what shall I do?" I recall confiding in my mother and other loved ones and all they could say was, "she's too young and too smart to be shackled with a baby, and you're too burdened down now to have to go through a pregnancy and have a baby to take care of afterwards." Eventually, with great concern, I conferred with her father, and all he could do was cry and tell me he would go along with whatever decision I made.

Growing up in the so-called ghetto of Chicago, I experienced, personally, the hardships, burdens and stigmas placed on the young unwed teenage mothers of my acquaintance. They were considered adult women and were not allowed to associate with girls their own age; nor were they allowed to attend day school. In addition, they were deemed loose and were scorned by the community.

All these things went through my mind as I sought to make, and did finally, make a decision to have the baby aborted. I do not remember asking Lydia what she wanted, but she assures me I did consult her. I remember asking her older sister where a clinic was where she could receive an abortion. Her older sister, living at that time in Kalamazoo, researched and found a clinic.

We made an appointment and followed through with the abortion. Later, I agonized about that decision; not knowing how it would affect Lydia, until a few years ago when she phoned me to discuss her long lasting depression, and the emotional state she was left in as a result of my decision. We never discussed it after she healed. However, I knew in my inner-most being that not allowing that child a chance to be born was contrary to my belief system. So when Lydia decided to discuss it with me, I was relieved, and with great humility asked her forgiveness. I had already made my peace with God.

You might ask if I had it to do over again, would I make the same decision. I would answer, if all factors were the same, including my ignorance of the emotional trauma that would be caused by that decision, yes. I have learned through the years that decisions made at any given time are based on many factors: emotional, mental, and physical needs, the degree of fear and stress, life's personal experiences, and that particular space in time.

I have also learned through this experience and other lessons of life, that when we sow, we must be prepared to reap the harvest thereof. But the wonderful thing about the sowing and the reaping is that when we recognize that after the planting lessons have been learned and we have struggled through the sowing and the dry, rainy and stormy seasons, we can, with joy, reap an abundant harvest. God smiled on both Lydia and me and blessed us with 5 wonderful children and grandchildren.

Now the rest of that old favorite song comes to mind: "He (Jesus the Christ) touched me, and oh the joy that floods my soul. Something happened, and now I know, He touched me and made me WHOLE!"

ooooo

After my mom discovered my suspected pregnancy, she took me to the doctor for a pregnancy test to confirm it. I still held out hope that I was not pregnant, but the test was positive. The lead coat of shame got a little heavier because now our family doctor, whose patient I had been for years, knew what I had done.

I still remember the drive home from the doctor's office. I felt like I was in a dream; this could not be happening to me. And for what? Because of one moment of stupidity on my part? More numbness.

As days dragged on, I still saw the agony on

my mom's face, but I figured she was agonizing over the fact that I was pregnant at fifteen and how a baby might negatively impact my life. I didn't know that, in addition to what I thought, she was agonizing over whether I would even have the baby. As I said in the introduction, abortion was not discussed like it is today. That option never entered my mind.

I, on the other hand, was trying to formulate a plan for how I could save my parents and myself embarrassment by leaving and having the baby somewhere else. I had a best friend in Chicago with whom I still kept in touch periodically. Her mother liked me, so I thought I would go live with them and have the baby, not telling anyone I was there. I then concluded that I could not bear to be away from my family, and leaving home without telling my parents would devastate them. They had experienced enough hurt because of me, so this plan was shelved.

My boyfriend and I discussed how we could possibly take care of the baby. We also talked with another couple in our school that had a baby. They explained how parenthood had changed them, their lives, and how they were managing it all. The young mother briefly described the symptoms of pregnancy and what would happen with my body. Of course, my body was already going through changes - one being my thickening abdomen that caused my clothes to fit snugly around my waist.

With each passing day, I grew more accustomed to the idea of being a mother. I loved taking care of children, and had accumulated plenty experience caring for my niece and nephew. I believed I could handle it.

Decision Day

The day came when I was informed of the decision. My mom and I sat in the living room of our small three-bedroom house.

"There is a way we can bring your period down," my mom said with a pained look on her face. I was excited and amazed we could do that. I didn't ask questions, but I wondered how that would happen. She told me my oldest sister knew of a clinic not far from our home that could do it.

My mind began processing what she said. *No period means pregnant, and period means not pregnant. If my period comes down, that will mean I am not pregnant any more. So, I am not going to have this baby, and I am not going to be a mother?* My mom was not one to be indecisive, and what she said, she meant, so it looked like this was pretty much settled. However, I had something to say, and I was wrestling with whether I should say it. Upsetting my mother more than I already had was something I had no desire to do, but I had to say it.

Hesitantly and without looking at her I said, "I want to have the baby." Her outward reaction did not give any indication that my comment had disturbed her. She only responded, "How are you going to take care of a baby?" Well, I had thought about this. "My boyfriend and I can get married, and he can work." This statement induced a chuckle that resonated with the message, "That's ridiculous." Although she did not actually say it was ridiculous, she made the point when she shot questions back at me like, "Are you both going to drop out of school?" "Where are you going to live?" "How is he going to find a job at his age to support all of you?"

That plan quickly went down the toilet. Before I brought up this option, I knew it was weak, but I had to try. I wanted to figure out a way to have the baby. However, because I truly had no idea how things were going to work out if I had the baby, I let it go. I just let it go. Thank goodness my anesthesia was still working pretty well at this point, or the disappointment would have made me curl up and cry.

The phone call was made to schedule the appointment. I was going to be about 12 weeks pregnant on the day my period would come down.

The term "abortion" was never mentioned, but at some point I must have realized that "bringing down my period" meant having an abortion.

Thanks to my anesthesia, life rolled on as usual.

chapter 5

It's Over, Right?

The day finally arrived. The "problem" was about to be taken care of. My mom, my sister and I got in the car early one spring morning to make our way to the clinic about 45 miles west of our home. We told the rest of the family we were going shopping. I am sure that must have seemed odd, since my mom was missing a day of work, and I was missing a day of school just to shop. Nevertheless, that was our alibi.

From the time I got in the car to the time I actually went into the room where the procedure took place, I was in a fog. It was surreal. Now I understand my mind was supplying the anesthetic necessary to endure this unnatural procedure.

At the clinic, I vaguely recall my mother

filling out the forms and then passing them to me to fill in the personal information about my last period, birth control, and other items. A lady then called me into a stark, little room where, some would say, she "counseled" me. I recall her asking me a few questions, and then she said a couple of things. Whatever she said could not have been very thorough, though, because I did not emerge from that room any more enlightened about what was going to happen than when I went in. Afterward, I sat back down with my mother and sister until I was called for the procedure.

I was taken to a large room with a changing area and another area where the procedure would take place. I was given instructions on how to put on the gown and where to put my clothes, and a reminder that I would need to wear a sanitary napkin when it was over.

Up to this point, I had been an emotionless automaton, mechanically following instructions on what to do and where to go. As I started to undress, however, tears, seemingly with a mind of their own, broke through the emotional numbness and began to roll down my cheeks. Right on their heels, came feelings of fear and loneliness. Either my emotional anesthesia was wearing off or there really could be no way to go through something like this and not feel anything. After I donned the gown, I sat on a bench in the large, empty room and waited - weeping, afraid, and alone.

A male doctor and a female nurse finally came in. Not one of their physical features imprinted in my memory. Once I left the room, they became faceless figures recognizable only by their positions at the table and their distinct attitudes.

The doctor told me to get on the table and put my feet in the stirrups. *Stirrups? Isn't that what cowboys use for their feet when riding a horse?* As I mounted the table, I saw two metal attachments protruding from its two end corners. *Ah, those must be the stirrups.* The nurse took her position by the right side of my head, and I could see the doctor at the foot of the table. Once my feet were in the stirrups, I was instructed to slide my bottom toward the edge of the table.

Oh, my God! This forward slide made my legs spread farther apart! I had never exposed myself to anyone like this before (except my boyfriend, of course). I was now lying on a table with my legs wide open exposing my private parts to a stranger - a man at that. More shame, more humiliation, and more tears.

The doctor told me I would feel some pain, and the nurse took my hand and told me to squeeze hers if I needed to. I was taken back by this kind gesture. It felt like someone had thrown me a lifeline just as I was about to drown in loneliness and despair. I did not just hold her hand, but I clung to the small bit of compassion she offered me. Whether it was genuine or just part of the routine, I did not know, but it kept me from going under.

In the background, I remember hearing a noise, something like a motor; then I felt the pain. Lots of pain. My weeping turned into loud wailing. The nurse tried to calm me down as I clutched her hand for dear life. I looked down so I could see what the doctor was doing, but the sheet covering my legs blocked my view. What was going on?

I am and always have been the kind of person who is not content with just knowing "what," I also need to know "why." So my mind quickly began working through the "why" behind this pain and the stress and strain of the past few weeks. The answer swiftly unfolded. It was because I had sex. Plain and simple. In a matter of seconds, I had weighed the "pleasure" of sex against my present ordeal and concluded the sex was hardly worth it; so in the midst of the procedure, I shouted, "I will never have sex again." Both the doctor and nurse chuckled, and to my surprise, the doctor said, "Oh, yes you will." I expected that he, an adult, would have encouraged me, a child, to refrain from having sex until I was older or married, but he didn't. For some reason, that made me angry.

When he finished, he told me I could get dressed, and he and the nurse promptly left the room. On to the next patient, I guessed. His apparent insensitivity and detachment from what he had done made me feel insignificant, like a nobody. But little did I know the worst was yet to come.

The "Recovery" Room

After I got dressed, I was escorted to a small room for a brief recovery period. There were about five other women there who were "recovering" from their abortions, as well. Did I mention this room was small? I sat in a recliner with my feet elevated and was offered orange juice and a cookie. *(It has just dawned on me, as I am writing this, that my "moment of truth" took place as I sat in a recliner with my feet up. Wow. I have come full circle.)*

I sat in that recliner sipping my juice, nibbling on my dry cookie, and sobbing like a baby. The other women sat with their juice and cookie in hand. A couple of them were weeping, and others just sat there stoically, all of us trying to avoid eye contact.

The memories of the recovery room are as painful as the abortion itself, perhaps more. I cannot adequately describe the embarrassment and humiliation of being forced to sit in what ended up as a circle in a small room, face to face with other people who now knew I had aborted.

We were all sitting there struggling, desperately trying to come to grips with what had just happened. This really should have been a private moment, but we had no privacy. It was horrible and inhumane. I and my pain were on display. It was like my privates were being exposed all over again. Another layer of shame and humiliation, another layer of anger.

Going Home

Once the "recovery" period ended, my mom, my sister and I got back in the car and headed home. Still crying, I told them what the doctor said about having sex. They laughed.

The day's events had me returning home with more shame than I had left with that morning, so I really was not looking forward to facing my dad. I could not handle another disgusted, disappointed look. After my mom parked the car in the garage, I exited and slowly made my way up the steps to the door. When I reached the landing, my dad was standing just inside the house holding the door open. I will never forget what happened next.

As I started walking past him with shame forcing me to look down so I would not have to see his face, he did something I did not expect. He reached out, grabbed me, and pulled me into his arms. He hugged me. He never said a word; he just hugged me. We stood there embracing, both of us crying. Nothing he could have said with his lips would have spoken love more eloquently to me than this hug. He still loved me, he still accepted me, and he empathized with the trauma I had just experienced. Although my father was close to death many times, I thank God that He kept him alive if for nothing more than this moment. My dad gave me something I needed - love and understanding - and I soaked up every bit like a dry sponge soaking up water. This would be the only consolation I would receive for the next twenty years.

My dad died a few months later. We enjoyed good times, as well as suffered bad times, but this memory of him stands out from the rest, and I will cherish it for the rest of my life.

After my dad released me from his comforting embrace, I drug myself to my bedroom and lay on the bed. I needed to pull myself together for school the next day. Regardless of the devastation that took place on this particular day, life had to go on. No one could know about it, so I had to put up a good front and pretend nothing happened. After all, I had only gone on a shopping trip.

I lay there for the rest of the day shutting down emotions until I was sufficiently numb. I didn't feel anything - not anger, not sadness, not loneliness, not anything. By the next day, I was "good to go." It was over . . . right?

chapter 6

Beginning the Healing
by Feeling the Pain

Now let's fast forward to my "moment of truth" almost twenty-two years later, as described in the first chapter. It is crystal clear that the abortion was far from over that day. Although I had "moved on with life," numb to the pain, anger, and shame of the abortion, those emotions had not gone away. They were just deeply buried, stashed away, yet inconspicuously causing major havoc in other areas of my life. (This havoc is detailed in Chapter 9).

After deciding I would deal with whatever was on the verge of erupting at a later time, I pulled myself together and continued with the rest of the evening as normally as I could.

The next day, Sunday, my husband and children and I prepared to go to church, despite the intense feelings of inner brokenness I was experiencing. I have seen other people skip worship services when they were going through difficult times, and I guess I could have stayed home also because this definitely qualified as a difficult time. However, in my many years of knowing Christ, I have learned that when hard times come, I *must* press my way into the house of God. It is in the praises of His people that He manifests His life-giving presence and ministers strength and peace to me through the music, fellowship and the preaching of His Word. On this particular Sunday, He met me once again.

The Word Was Already Prepared

The service began with songs of praise and worship led by my husband, who was the Minister of Music. Peace flooded my soul as we entered the Lord's presence through anointed songs of worship. My emotions remained in check for the rest of the service - that is until the time came to hear the ministry of the Word.

My pastor was out of town, so one of the women on our ministerial staff preached. She announced the Lord was leading her to minister on the subject of healing the hurts of the past.

I sat there stunned. How did she know the hurts of my past had just been resurrected from some deep, dark, cryptic place? Then I came to myself and realized that the Lord was allowing me to see what He's shown me over and over again; when He reveals something that's difficult to handle, it is not so I can feel bad, but it is so He can heal it. God had revealed the abortion as the root of my pain the night before, and I definitely felt bad, but He would not let it rest until He healed it. Out of His unending love and compassion, He meticulously planned the catalyst, time, and setting for my healing. He is the Master Planner.

As the woman of God preached about how the Lord wants us to live free from the pain of our past, I felt like I was the only person in the room to whom the Lord was speaking. I sensed His Spirit gently urging me to release my pain, but I was sitting on the platform with the other ministers at the front of the church in full view of the congregation, so I tried to hold back. I still did not know specifically what was in me trying to surface, and its intensity the night before had frightened me. It took everything in me not to burst into tears.

The preacher continued, saying the Lord wanted us to be whole, so we had to stop avoiding our pain and allow Him to heal it. I could not hold it in any longer. The tears began to flow. I tried to be inconspicuous as I silently cried and wiped the tears from my face.

After the message, she asked those who wanted special prayer for healing to come to the altar. I desperately needed prayer, but I did not have the strength to stand up and walk down from the platform to the altar, so I just rested my head on my lap.

As I sat there, I suddenly got a strange sensation in my genitals. Compulsively, I pressed my thighs together tighter and tighter. Actually, I had a strong urge to put my hand over my vagina in the same way someone would put their hand over a body part that had just been injured. It did not hurt, but something painful had taken place. Violation.

The dictionary defines violation as "desecration, infringement, intrusion," and this perfectly describes what I felt at that moment. A strong sense of violation seemed to be flowing through my veins from the top of my head to the soles of my feet, seeping through the pores of my skin. I felt desecrated, intruded and infringed upon.

It was obvious something was wrong with me, and out of concern, one of the elders approached me and tenderly laid his hand on my shoulder. Although I am normally the "touchy-feely queen" and thrive on touches, his touch was repulsive to me, so I jerked away. Others came to minister to me, but I would not let them touch me either. I felt like I could not stand it.

One of the ladies asked me what was going on, and through my sobs, all I could say was, "The abortion . . ." I had known this particular sister for many years, and she was aware the Lord had delivered me in other abortion-related areas years before, so she said, "Haven't you already received ministry for this?" The way she said it gave me the impression she thought I should have been over the abortion by now. That thought had crossed my mind, too, but through this and other experiences I and women I have ministered to have had, I have learned that *time does not heal all wounds.* Whoever said it does, lied. The wounds may burrow deeper and deeper in the soul or spirit; or we may deny we have wounds, but the truth is, we are not healed until we are healed.

While still sobbing, I responded to her and said, "No, this is different. This is different." I was doubled over, and probably looked like I was in pain, but the pain wasn't physical.

Facing the Pain

When we are wounded, many times we take the pain, put it in a closet somewhere in our heart or mind, shut the door, lock it, and throw away the key. We do not ever want to feel it or deal with it again. While that may be our way of dealing with pain, it is definitely not God's. He says in Isaiah 55:8, "For my thoughts are not your thoughts, neither are your ways my ways . . ." (KJV)

You see, when we lock away our pain, it isn't gone, it isn't healed; it's just out of sight, or more accurately, "out of touch." We think because we don't feel anything, we must be okay.

Jehovah Rapha, the Lord our healer, however, is not content with us walking around wounded, but unable to feel the pain. In the physical body, this is a dangerous phenomenon. If your body is hurt, and you can't feel the pain, you are missing out on the distress signal that tells your brain, "I need help!"

My dad is a perfect example. He was partially paralyzed on his right side and had little feeling in his right leg. One of the few things he could do was cut grass because he could sit on our riding lawn mower. His right foot sat by the motor, and because it took him a while to cut the grass (we had five acres of land), the motor grew very hot. One day, the heat from the motor badly burned his foot, but he did not realize it until after he had come into the house and saw it with his eyes.

We numb ourselves to emotional pain, like my dad's foot was numb to the physical pain, but the fact remains we are wounded, just like my dad's foot was wounded. Serious wounds do not heal by themselves. Without proper treatment, they tend to get worse and can affect or infect other areas.

Many of us are wounded, but unable to deal with the pain that is locked in the closet. We're thinking we're okay because we don't feel anything. However, we can't sleep at night, we fly into rages at the drop of a hat, we cry about little things, we can't get close to people, we are sick much of the time, we suffer from depression - it manifests in many ways. We're not okay. The Lord doesn't want us numb, He wants us healed, and He wants us whole.

In Jeremiah 8:10, God was displeased with the spiritual leaders of that day because they were not truthful with the people. Rather, they were misleading them. He says in verse 11, "For they have healed the hurt of the daughter of my people slightly, saying, Peace, peace, when there is no peace." (KJV)

In many of our lives, we have mistaken numbness for peace. Thus, we are saying peace, peace, but there is really no peace.

Life is in the Blood

My dad had also developed a condition called arteriosclerosis (hardening of the arteries), which severely hindered the flow of blood to his foot. The lack of blood flowing to his foot impaired his foot's ability to heal. Thus, the sore grew worse.

Leviticus 17:11 states, "The life of the flesh is in the blood . . ." The blood flowing freely through our bodies brings life to all its members. When arteries and veins are blocked, the blood that carries life cannot flow, and *de*generation takes place. Body parts deteriorate and wither just like my dad's foot.

With emotional and spiritual hurts locked away, they are cut off from the life-giving blood that Jesus shed for us. There is power in His blood to save, heal, and deliver us. He poured out His blood, His life, so we could live. Not just be alive, but really live. He died so we could be *re*generated.

It is difficult to open the closet door and expose our pain, but this is the first stop on the path to wholeness. We must be willing to open the door to the emotions that have been blocked, so the blood of Jesus can flow to them, bringing regeneration, health and wholeness.

Reliving the Abortion

In obedience to the Lord's prompting the night before and through this timely Sunday message, I began opening closet doors that had sealed off the emotional and spiritual pain of my abortion 22 years before.

While still on the platform at my church, the Lord led me back to the room where the abortion took place, and it felt as if I was going through it all over again. This time, however, I was reliving it with a clearer understanding of what was happening. Although I had numbed myself emotionally the first time, this time, I felt everything. It was difficult, but in it, the Lord was revealing to me the truth about the abortion and the emotional distress it caused.

Another woman in ministry asked me to follow her into a room where she and a couple of other people would continue ministering to me. When we got there, she asked me to explain what was happening. I told her I now realized that the abortion was a violation of my body, and I was actually feeling the violation. I cried, "The doctor went into *my* body and took *my* baby. He violated me! It was like he raped me!" Once I verbalized it, the suppressed anger began to rise. I was very, very angry with the doctor. The understanding of what he did, along with my resurfaced memory of the callousness in which he did it, made me livid.

The Connection between Mother and Son

In verbally describing the violation, I heard myself connect the words *my* and *baby* for the first time. *My baby*. Although I knew, even at fifteen, that a baby, not just a blob of tissue, had been aborted, I never connected with the truth that the baby was *my* baby. I had never connected with the baby as *my* son. Maybe emotionally disconnecting from him was a way for me to cope with the loss. Whatever the reason, I know that 22 years later, I became that baby's mother, and that baby became my son.

I never saw him, but I have always known in my heart he was a boy. I was a mother who had lost a son - a son who would have then been 21 years old. This revelation was almost too much to bear.

Loneliness

The Lord had broken the emotional dam, so more emotions began to emerge.

All of a sudden, I felt an overwhelming sense of loneliness. I do not remember ever feeling this lonely. Feelings of loneliness were present at the abortion, but I must have been somewhat numb because I had not felt them to this degree. In my mind, I saw myself in the abortion room sitting alone, crying, fearful of what was about to take place. The picture was so clear. The feelings were so strong. Why was no one there with me? Why was I going through this by myself?

In asking myself these questions, I was not solely addressing the issue of sitting alone in the room - no, there was more to it. The loneliness stemmed from the fact that there was no one, not just in the room, but *with me* emotionally; there was no one empathetic to the trauma I was suffering.

Diana Ross, the singer, would ask her audience a question when she performed: "Can you feel me?" She wanted to know if the audience was connecting with the emotions she felt as she sang a particular song.

Well, there was no one who "felt me." No one connected to the fear and insecurity of a fifteen-year-old child who had no idea how to effectively handle the drama of abortion. There was no one to help me along in the process. That's why my dad's actions after I returned home were so valuable. Over a twenty or so year period, he was the only one who demonstrated any signs of "feeling me."

I never thought of loneliness as pain, but as I sat in church reliving that fateful day, the pain of that loneliness pierced me down to the core. It's no wonder I numbed it. I, as an adult, began to grieve for the child I saw in the room.

The Affirmation I Needed

I continued to verbally express to those ministering to me the emotions that were surfacing like popcorn popping. One sister wisely and lovingly validated whatever I felt. For instance, when I said

I was violated, she said, "Yes, you were." I needed someone to see and understand that. If she had said, "No, don't feel that way" or "you shouldn't feel like that," I think the emotional flow would have been cut off, and I would have closed up, feeling like maybe I was just being irrational. I thank God for that sister's sensitivity to the Spirit of God in how to help me. She did not discount what I felt, but affirmed it, and this gave me the freedom and courage to continue facing whatever surfaced.

My sisters in Christ prayed for me as the Spirit led them, but they knew and I knew that I was not going to be completely healed at that time. I had buried and carried these things for years, and it would take time to dig and sort through it all. The Lord had purposed to heal me, not slightly, but thoroughly.

God Uses People

As the women of God brought the time of ministry to a close, they gave me scriptures on which to meditate as I continued my healing journey. I thank God for my brothers and sisters in Christ, especially those in my own local church. They have always been a source of comfort and encouragement in my times of distress, and this time was no different. There is a heavy cloak of shame that covers post-abortive women, and for me, it was and still is an enormous blessing to have spiritual brothers and sisters to whom I can expose what I have done without being judged and condemned. They truly love me with God's unconditional love. When they look at me they do not see the sin I committed, but they see me as a woman of God and still eagerly receive the ministry God has given me.

The Lord does not want us to go through our trials alone. He says in Romans 15:1, "the strong ought to bear the infirmities of the weak" (KJV). Many of us have trouble with this concept because we do not want to admit that we are weak in certain areas. We have to believe that "we are strong," and "we can handle it." The way we end up handling it, however, is through self-anesthetization or denial, and because we don't feel pain, we believe we are strong. Real strength manifests when we can confront our painful experiences and allow God to bring true healing.

We also have difficulty because we see ourselves as independent - we don't need anyone. Then there are those who just don't want anyone else to know their struggles for fear of rejection. Actually, the root of these issues is pride. It takes humility to admit, "I can't handle this on my own. I'm not strong enough to deal with it. I'm going to get help, regardless of what people think of me. I trust God."

As I will discuss later, carrying our burdens alone only serves to make problems worse. God sends people in our lives that will demonstrate His mercy and love to us and help us in our seasons of weakness. Many times we want God, in His sovereignty, to help us, and at times He will, but He also chooses to use people as vessels of His loving-kindness, mercy and healing.

Throughout the 22 years prior to my moment of truth, the Lord had healed me of other abortion-related issues. He would connect something I was dealing with to the abortion, and then show me how to deal with it, which was mostly through prayers for deliverance. This particular time, I had no idea how to handle it. I needed help.

chapter 7

Laying the Axe to the Root

The next day, I lay sprawled face down on my living room floor crying out to God, "Help me, I can't deal with this alone. It's too much for me. I don't know what to do." This was the first time in my 36 years I remember feeling this helpless and overwhelmed. I imagine this is how David felt when he wrote Psalms 61:1–2:

> *Hear my cry, O God; attend unto my prayer.*
> *From the end of the earth will I cry unto thee,*
> *when my heart is overwhelmed; lead me to the*
> *rock that is higher than I. (KJV)*

The exact location of the end of the earth referenced in this verse is a mystery to me, but I cried to God dangling from the end of myself and my self-help abilities. And He heard my cry. He picked me up and led me to a place that was higher than I, and what I could do in my own strength. He spoke to me by His Spirit and said, "Get up, go get the newspaper and look for a support group." Once again, I knew this was without a doubt the Lord speaking because I would have never come up with that idea on my own.

At the time, my city's newspaper published lists of various community organizations and their meeting times on the first Sunday of the month. When I found the newspaper, I looked inside, and it just so happened to be that particular edition. There were seemingly hundreds of groups listed for various needs like alcoholism, abuse, widows, singles, and so on. In desperation, I ran my finger down every listing until I came across a section for post-abortion. The term "post-abortion" was new to me, but I figured because I was seeking help "after" an abortion, it applied to me. There was one group listed and because the phone number was the only information given, I could not tell whether the group was Christian. Under normal circumstances, I would have sought a Christian group, but I was in such distress, it did not matter.

I called the number, and my emotional mix of excitement and anxiety sank to disappointment as an automated voice responded to my call. The voice informed me I had reached the Pregnancy Counseling Center. I had driven by this center hundreds of times, but I was unsure whether or not it was an abortion clinic. Out of despair and in obedience to the Lord, I left a message asking someone to call me with more information.

Now to Him...

Time must have slipped into some "super slow-mo" realm because minutes passed like hours as I anxiously awaited a return call. This phenomenon happened only once before in my life - the day my father died. That day, a Sunday, was without question the longest day of my life. I was certain some kind of natural law existed extending daylight in the summer and shortening it in the winter; but it was December, for goodness sake, and night seemed to take its own sweet time showing up. I just wanted the day to be over so I could go to bed and slip into unconsciousness for a while. (Ah, sleep - the other anesthetic.) It was torment.

I was being tormented again. Although my call was returned the same day, it felt like days had passed. The lady who called me back was named Mary. She said she did not know if I was a Christian, but I should know the post-abortion group was a Bible study led by Christian women. I could have passed out. I would have accepted any kind of help at that point, but the Lord knew when He told me to look in the paper that the group was Christian and Bible-based. I began to cry. Actually, I sobbed... audibly. As Mary continued to talk over my sobs, I sensed she was accustomed to this sort of emotional response - it must have happened often.

Mary explained how the Lord moves in the group and shared testimonies of how women had been healed. The icing on the cake was when she said that at the end of the Bible study, there would be a memorial service for the babies. I could name my baby, and in that service, I would be given the opportunity to give him a special tribute.

This was too much for me; almost too good to be true. My heart leaped for joy at the thought that my baby would have a name, an identity, and I would be able to do something special for him. The group was turning out to be more than I could have imagined. I have a personal, experiential knowledge of Ephesians 3:20 which says:

> *Now to him who is able to do immeasurably more than all we ask or imagine according to his power that is at work in us. (NIV)*

The "him" referred to here is God the Father, and my expectations were being immeasurably exceeded!

Needless to say, I was ready to sign up. Show me the dotted line! "When does it start?" I asked, hoping she would say tomorrow. Instead, she said the leaders of the group preferred to have a minimum number of women participate, so I had to wait for a few more women to sign up. She did not know how long that would take. It was December, but she was hoping to start the first of February at the earliest. *"February?!"*

I felt my heart beginning its descent into disappointment once again. Would someone please get me off this rollercoaster? Before it hit bottom, the Lord gently reminded me that He had ordained this for me, and He would keep me until the group started. I felt myself leveling off.

In the Meantime

Shortly after making contact with the Pregnancy Counseling Center, I began having dreams about the baby's father. Many years had passed since I had seen him, but for some reason, he held a recurring role in my dreams.

In the dreams, an urgent need to talk with him drove me on a frantic search to find him; but he always eluded me. I would literally run to his mother's home hoping he would be there, only to be told he was at his sister's; then upon arriving at his sister's home, I would learn I had just missed him. I would see him walking down the street, and after anxiously running to catch up with him, disappointment would strike once again as the person turned out to be someone else.

I am rarely able to recall the dreams that invade my sleep almost every night, but upon awakening after these, I not only remembered them, but the intense frustration with my inability to talk to him lingered; so I knew these dreams held significant meaning. Irritated, I would lie in bed questioning myself and God, "Why do I need to talk to this man?"

I surely was not yearning to talk with him in reality. After my last encounter with him about twelve years before, I concluded it would be no great loss if I never saw him again. At the time, he, like I, was married, and on my way home from a visit with my mother, who lived in the same town as he, I decided to pay him a visit. We had been very close, not just as lovers, but as friends for most of my teen years, so I was interested in how he was doing.

As I rang the doorbell to his apartment, a subtle current of anxiety rippled through me. It had been a few years since I had talked with him, and I did not know what to expect. He opened the door and appeared to be sincerely happy to see me.

I took a seat on the living room sofa in the bright, spacious, and airy apartment, while he took a seat at the opposite end. We were having a pleasant conversation when out of nowhere, he abruptly changed the topic of our discussion to the abortion. He didn't say much, but I was light years away from being able to handle what he did say. I immediately decided it was time for me to leave. Thus, I responded, "It's time for me to go." I got up, said my goodbyes, and left.

While in the bed after one of the dreams, that long-ago conversation popped into my mind. As I reflected on how the tremendous surge of emotions stemming from the abortion had crippled me in recent weeks, I was able to look at what he said in a new, brighter light. This light illuminated his pain. It dawned on me that he, like me, was hurting from the loss of his child.

From somewhere within my spirit, a question arose, "Did you and he ever discuss the abortion?" We continued to date at least two years after the abortion, so I was certain we had. However, as I strained to recall any discussion between us, nothing materialized. I suddenly realized the baby's father and I *never* talked about the abortion or the baby after it was over. Never. I was flabbergasted. How could that have happened?

I was fifteen and he was sixteen, soon to be seventeen, when we lost the baby, and I guess maybe we were too young to understand and work through it on our own. I Corinthians 13:11 says,

> When I was a child, I talked like a child, I thought like a child, I reasoned like a child. When I became a man, I put childish ways behind me. (NIV)

It became clear to me that because we were both children at the time of the abortion, our understanding and thoughts about it were immature. However, when we became adults, we developed an adult's understanding of this tragic event. It was also clear that his understanding matured much quicker than mine.

He had abruptly brought up the abortion out of his own sense of loss and pain. Generally, the emotions of the fathers of aborted babies are not considered with any amount of concern, and because no one had reached out to help me heal, I was certain he had not received any assistance either. For his words to burst out so suddenly, the baby must have been on his mind and heart for some time. Now, I not only hurt for my baby and me, I hurt for him, too.

Could our last abruptly began and abruptly ended conversation be seeking resolution and closure by pushing me in that direction through my dreams? Unsure of the next step, I decided to wait and see how God would lead me through the group.

The dreams persisted.

Grief

One night, as I sat in a Sunday evening service at my church, I felt sadness slowly creep up on me like a dark shadow in a mystery movie. My mind wandered away from the worship service, and I began to think about my son. Tears once again poured from my eyes as I thought about how I would never see him, hug him, or hold him. I was sitting in the back of the church this time, so only the person sitting next to me saw my tears. She was my best friend, and even though I knew she was concerned, thankfully, she was sensitive enough to discern it was not the time for questions or comfort. I wanted to be left alone, and without a word between us, she complied.

I was tired of crying, and a little nagging voice kept whispering in my ear, "Why don't you just get over it? You're being ridiculous. You're making a big deal out of nothing. You were not even pregnant that long. You can't be that attached." Half-believing it, I drug myself to the bathroom to blow my nose. I looked at myself in the mirror. Totally disgusted with my red eyes and nose, I scolded my reflection, "Lydia, you have to pull yourself together. You can't keep crying like this all the time. You are such a wuss." Falling back into the "shut it down, so you can appear strong" mode, I stuffed the sadness down until it felt in check. I took a deep breath, threw my shoulders back and returned to my seat in the sanctuary. Slowly, thoughts about my lost son made their way back into the forefront of my mind. My shoulders drooped in tandem with my drooping resistance. Sadness overtook me again.

Exasperated, I asked the Lord what was going on. What was this? He answered, "Grief." He explained that I had never grieved the loss of my child. It was the sadness that occurs after a loved one dies, and you realize you will never see that person again. He is forever absent from your life. Even though I was sitting in a worship service, I felt like I was at a funeral - my son's funeral.

I hurt. My arms throbbed, aching with an unfulfilled longing to hold him. I felt empty, but also sensed the familiar heaviness in my chest. Feelings of nausea rolled in my stomach; I wanted to throw up.

No one ever told me I could or should grieve for him. I guess the folks at the clinic did not tell me because to them, he was not a person; they wouldn't think grieving was necessary. I, and apparently no one else involved, understood that grieving is appropriate when a child dies through abortion before he/she is born. It is interesting, however, that this concept is embraced in the termination of a baby's life through miscarriage. I had seen support groups and information galore on emotional healing because of miscarriage, but none for the loss of a child through abortion.

While still sitting in the back of the church, I drooped to the point where my head once again laid on my lap. Slowly, a picture materialized in my mind like a still photo developing in a darkroom. In the picture, I saw a young man dressed in a white suit standing with his hand in his pant pocket looking very suave. The background of the picture hinted he may have been at a formal party. Although I could not see distinct facial features, he resembled my oldest son - his skin was light and hair dark. In my heart, I knew it was him - the son I had lost. The Lord, out of His mercy, had given me a picture.

The only way I can describe my feelings in this moment is to paint another picture. Imagine a child who never knew her parents because they died when she was a baby. She longs to know more about them - how they looked, their likes and dislikes, their personalities, anything. After years have passed and the curiosity has turned into a nagging ache of incompletion, a family friend sees her sorrow, and says, "I have a picture of your parents, and I want you to have it." She's overjoyed and can hardly believe she's finally going to have something tangible of her long-lost loved ones, even if it is just a glimpse of their faces at one moment in time. Her parents finally move from being some sort of legendary tale to people with faces with whom she can identify. She coddles and treasures the picture, pulls it out and looks at it longingly when she thinks of her parents, wondering how her life would have been if they had lived. She finds consolation in troubled times by softly stroking her parents' faces or holding the picture close to her chest.

This was me with the picture of my son. The Lord was my family friend who knew I was at a point when I needed and could handle something "tangible" of my son. Some post-abortive women picture their children forever as infants, some as toddlers, and some see them at the age they would be at the time they are thinking of them. I saw my son at the age he would have been then, 21.

The aching of my empty arms continued for weeks, but I had the consolation of closing my eyes, pulling out that picture and stroking his face with fleshless hands and holding it against a fleshless chest.

The Gift of My Husband

At times, when I am attacked with doubts about whether God really loves me, I only look at my husband, and I see the Lord's boundless love for me. I thank God continually for giving me Tim. He is my gift. Every now and then, the other men who proposed marriage come to mind, and I have to shake my head. It is not that they were bad men, but when I reflect on the drama my husband has endured over the years because of my issues, I know they would not have been able to stick it out with me. Tim truly loves me unconditionally, and he does not get bent out of shape about the emotional ups and downs I have suffered because of the abortion. He just listens, and does whatever he can to help me heal.

One night, as we were lying in the bed talking, I shared with Tim my sense of loss and sadness because I would never get to see, hold, or know my baby. He then responded to me in his laid back manner, "But you'll get to see him in heaven." I paused and pondered that for a second. The proverbial light bulb illuminated. Wow! He was right! How could I have missed that point? I would see my son when I got to heaven! Relief and comfort flooded me. There was hope. I looked at my husband and my heart overflowed once again with gratitude for him and to him. In addition to being right about what he said, it touched me that he really heard what I was saying, not just politely listening. He cared enough to hear God give him a word of truth that helped settle me.

Finally, the Group Begins

After impatiently waiting, the call announcing the start of the group finally came. A woman named Susan called and said she would be leading the group with an assistant, and she wanted to have a one-on-one session before it began to gather information about me. We scheduled the appointment for the preliminary meeting.

When I arrived at her house on the day of our appointment, I sat in her driveway for a moment, nervous, yet excited, and almost in disbelief that at last, I would finally have the opportunity, the place, and the people to work through the drama and trauma of the abortion.

I got out of the car, and as she had instructed on the phone, I knocked on the side door of her small ranch home. Susan, a petite lady in her fifties, opened the door and greeted me with a warm smile and hug that allayed any remnants of nervousness. As we walked down the stairs leading to her basement, she guaranteed that her husband, who was upstairs, would stay out of sight and hearing range.

We both sat down at a small table. She began by telling me a little about herself and the group. She then said she needed to ask me questions about myself and the abortion, and she assured me it would be okay if I could not answer some of the questions.

I began to cry, again. (How many tears could I possibly have left?) After gathering general information like my address and phone number, she began asking abortion-specific questions. As with Mary, I found comfort in the fact that my continual crying did not deter Susan from gently forging ahead with her task of collecting information. Her actions reassured me I was not crazy or over-emotional, but my reactions were normal.

On one of the questions, she explained that she was going to read a list of symptoms some women experience immediately after an abortion. After she read each symptom, I was to respond "yes" if I had experienced it immediately after my abortion or "no" if I had not. As we proceeded down the list of about 30 symptoms, I found myself answering yes to more than a few. Each time I uttered "yes" to behaviors and feelings that hounded me as a teen - like crying spells, suicidal thoughts, fear of failure, depression, and alcohol - another dot was connected and the picture became clearer that I had suffered these things as a result of the abortion! I had no idea.

It literally felt like the pieces of a puzzle were finally coming together forming a complete picture of the emotional suffering and resulting behaviors I experienced as a teen and young adult. Up to this point they had been random, pointless, isolated events; but now they were connected to something! What was more exciting was that I was now in a group that the Lord would use to heal and restore me. He was not just going to heal me now, but the healing was going to reach back more than twenty years.

In Joel 2:25, the Lord promises,

And I will restore to you the years that the locust hath eaten, the cankerworm, and the caterpillar, and the palmerworm, my great army which I sent among you. (KJV)

The Lord was going to restore the years of my life that had been eaten by depression, sorrow and alcohol.

Later in the interview, Susan went through the same list again, asking if I had experienced any of the symptoms in the past six months. I responded affirmatively to some of the same symptoms as the first time, but new ones had surfaced within the last six months, like the dreams/nightmares, regret, anger, panic feelings and sexual problems.

Earlier, I wrote of the process of self-anesthetization and how we lock away painful emotions and experiences. In order to cope with the trauma of the abortion, I did what I had to do to continue living. I reasoned with myself that it was over, so I completely blocked out any emotions related to that experience. I am and always have been emotional, but from that point, I made no connection between the abortion and any other negative emotion or behavior I exhibited. Now I realized the emotions had been blocked from my consciousness, but they were manifesting in other ways.

As we wrapped up the interview, Susan told me we were going to use the book *Forgiven and Set Free,* by Linda Cochrane for the Bible study. She gave me the book and told me to have the first lesson completed by the initial group session, which would begin on March 8.

The Lord had kept his promise to keep me from going over the edge for the two and a half month period between my moment of truth and the beginning of the group.

Telling My Mother about the Group

After moving away from home at age eighteen, my mom and I talked at least once a week. I was excited about the upcoming group, and I wanted to share this good news with her. However, she and I had not talked much about the abortion, and I could not predict her reaction.

When I was twenty-four, she came to my home to help me after the birth of my first child. Seeing my first-born baby must have triggered something in her because she brought up the abortion for the first time since the day it happened. We were sitting in the living room of my small apartment, and she was holding my son. I know it must have been difficult for her to bring it up, but she said, "Lydia, I just need to ask you to forgive me for making the decision for the abortion." I never had animosity against my mother for the decision she made because I believed she felt she had my best interest at heart. Because of that and the fact that I really did not want to deal with it at the time, I just waved my hand and said, "Oh, mom. I forgive you." "I hope so," she said. That was it.

As various issues related to the abortion manifested later in my adulthood, I never discussed them with her. This was mostly because I sensed she still struggled with guilt about making the decision, and I did not want her to come under any more condemnation knowing the abortion had negatively affected other areas of my life. At least one other time she brought up the abortion by saying, "I hope you have forgiven me for the abortion." Once again, I avoided any in-depth discussion about it, but reassured her I had.

Now to tell her that I would be going through this eight-week Bible study support group would be revealing that I had serious issues resulting from the abortion. I was risking making her feel bad, but leaving her out of this momentous occasion did not seem right. She was my mother, and I wanted her to be a part of what promised to be a major turn in my life. When I called, I kept it simple. I told her about the group and let her know I would be participating. She asked, "Why?" I explained, "The abortion messed me up in a lot of ways."

Her response caught me off guard. She said, "You're not over that yet! It happened so long ago, and you are still dealing with it?"

I love and respect my mom immensely, and I generally do not raise my voice at her or lose my temper, but her response and its tone pushed a button that caused me to explode. (This unknown button, which I will discuss later, was uncovered in the group.) I yelled, "Over it? How would I have gotten over it? No one said *anything* to me after the abortion. Not one word! I was 15 years old! How was I supposed to deal with it? I was a kid! Tell me mom, how would I have gotten over it?" As you can probably guess, I started crying.

The suddenness and intensity of my outburst startled me, so I am sure it must have startled my mom, also. I cannot recall what was said after that because from that point, my number one goal was to get off the phone. After we hung up, it took a while for me to gain my composure.

When the anger subsided, I looked again at what my mother said and why she probably said it. I know she loves me and would never intentionally hurt me, so I tried to understand her response. I concluded that to my mom, the fact that I was going through the group meant that I was still hurting from the abortion, and because the abortion was her decision, it meant her decision was still causing me pain. This pushed the button of guilt in her, like her response pushed the button of anger in me. (Although I anticipated my news stirring guilt in her, the way it manifested threw me off.)

After reaching this conclusion, I decided to talk to her as sparingly as possible about the group and whatever happened therein. I did not want to make her feel worse than she already did, and I certainly was in no condition to tactfully handle her responses. I must have adhered to that decision because she told me almost seven years later that I never shared with her the outcome of the group.

The First Meeting

I was excited, but nervous about the first meeting of the group. Like the intake interview, the meetings were held in Susan's basement. There were two other black post-abortive women in the group, and we were all from Pentecostal churches. If you know anything about black Pentecostal Christians, you know that we can be very *expressive* in our worship and prayers. Susan, on the other hand, was a soft-spoken Catholic white lady, and her assistant, Pat, was a soft-spoken Lutheran white lady.

This was my first experience receiving ministry from sisters in these segments of the body of Christ, and the anointing of the Lord rested heavily upon them. They were women of faith who constantly reassured us that God was going to meet us in the Bible study and heal us. They exhibited the compassion of our Lord - when we cried, they cried with us; they were neither judgmental nor condemning. We could sense their genuine concern for us and our babies, and they allowed the Lord to lead them as they led us through the Bible study.

I will not go over everything we discussed in the group, although it was ALL good. I will just highlight some of the things that impacted me the most.

The Root Exposed

In the first session, Susan asked us to draw a picture of our pain. We were to think about how our pain felt, how it might look, and draw it. She gave us paper, crayons, markers, and colored pencils to use and gave us some time to work. I am not an artist, but I knew exactly how to describe what I felt. I drew an outline of the front view of a person with their head turned to the side. In the center of its chest, I colored a large, black rectangular shape, which represented the heavy, icky feeling sitting in my chest. In the center of the abdomen, I drew a crude stomach attached to a tube that led from the stomach, through the black rectangle on the chest and up to my mouth. Lastly, I drew little spatters coming from the mouth representing the urge I had to throw up.

Next, Susan passed out a sheet of paper listing the group's guidelines, the group's purpose and task areas of healing. One purpose of the group was to experience forgiveness and one of the tasks was to deal with issues of guilt and accepting

God's forgiveness. Thankfully, I had received God's forgiveness years before. I had no doubt that the Lord was not holding the abortion against me. However, another purpose and task stood out for me - they dealt with grieving the loss of the child.

As Susan reviewed the handout, my eyes were constantly drawn to the statements about grief. My curiosity was stirred about this concept of "grieving my aborted child." I knew I was grieving because I felt the sadness, but I sensed it went deeper.

Susan began to explain how few post-abortive women are aware of the need to grieve their lost children. A woman who loses a child to miscarriage receives support and understanding for her loss, while women who abort do not, further supporting the deception that it is not appropriate to grieve.

Then, she gave us a handout entitled, "What Grief Looks Like." It described how grief affects us in five areas - emotionally, cognitively, physically, behaviorally and spiritually - and it gave a detailed list of symptoms in each category. As I read over the lists, the light bulb above my head illuminated once again. I got the revelation that a good portion of my emotional suffering over the past two decades was rooted in *unresolved grief.* In the intake interview, I got the connection between the abortion and certain symptoms I had experienced throughout my life; now their relationship to grief made the connection between the pain and the abortion more specific. Eureka!

Earlier in this chapter, I explained I was unaware of the need to grieve the loss of my child until the Lord revealed it to me while I sat in a church service. I then, at least, allowed myself to feel the pain of the loss of his precious life. Until this session, however, I did not understand the complexity of unresolved grief, and its impact on all areas of life. Now it was apparent that the seed of grief I had buried long ago grew into a tree that produced fruit of anger, depression, fatigue, upset stomach, frequent crying, nervousness, worry, preoccupation with death, inability to concentrate, suicidal thoughts, alcohol, self-blame, loneliness, and numbness. I was flabbergasted. For years, all I could see was the fruit; but now, finally, the root.

Jesus said in John 8:32, "And you shall know the truth, and the truth shall make you free." (KJV)

For me, just finally knowing the truth about what had me bound was liberating all by itself. It was also liberating to know it was not absurd to hurt and cry for a child I never knew. The Lord had revealed to me the need to grieve a few weeks before, but now that it had been confirmed, this truth was sealed in my heart, and I knew the devil would no longer be able to torment me with thoughts that my sorrow was unwarranted. I did not have to fight my feelings of sadness; I only had to work through it. Freedom, freedom!

The Labor

Susan encouraged us not to take on additional responsibilities for the duration of the Bible study; she said we needed time to complete the lessons each week and time to allow God to speak to us about them. She also told us that going through this process could be emotionally draining, so we should enlist support people who could help lighten our load and give us space to work through our issues.

Susan was certainly right because after each session, all I could do was go home and fall in my bed, thoroughly exhausted. I explained to *my* support person, my husband, what Susan said, and as usual, he came through. He handled the children and the household duties on the days I attended the sessions giving me the time I needed afterward to rest, regroup, and allow the Lord to continue His work in me.

There was one thing Susan and Pat often expressed to my fellow group members and me which was particularly comforting - "We know it is difficult to deal with your abortions like this. It takes a lot of courage to do what you are doing, and we admire and appreciate you for it." Yes, it was difficult, and although I had not considered it before, it did take a lot of courage. The questions in the Bible study made us think hard and dig through our self-deceptions, misconceptions, unforgiveness, anger, hurt and regret. It was painful and laborious, but as the saying goes, "no pain, no gain." I was willing to suffer the pain to gain restoration, peace, and wholeness.

My Baby's Daddy

In one of the sessions, I shared with the group the dreams I was having about finding the baby's daddy. I asked the women what they thought the dreams meant. They concluded the dreams probably meant I should talk with him, but I should definitely let the Holy Spirit lead me.

I prayed about it and sensed I should call him, but I would only do so with my husband's consent. I shared the dreams with Tim and told him I felt impressed to talk with the baby's daddy. He was hesitant because we had no idea how the baby's daddy would respond, and he did not want any more pain added to the load with which I was already struggling. However, he thought the dreams were a strong indication that I should call, so he consented.

I called information for the city in which I heard he lived, and they had a phone listing for him. I had to psych myself up to dial the number. As I sat on the edge of my bed looking at the phone, I felt like a trainer trying to stir a boxer to win a match as I told myself, "You can do this. It will be okay. Everything will be fine. You would not be having the dreams if this was not what you should be doing. You can do it; dial the number." After a couple of minutes, I was bouncing around my imaginary ring with my dukes up, ready to go. Pumped up, yet nervous, I dialed his phone number. After our last visit, I had no idea how he would receive my call, especially since I was calling to discuss the abortion. I mentally prepared myself for the worst, but in my heart, I believed it would be okay because I sensed the Lord was in it. The phone rang. Then it rang again . . . and again. He was not home. Arghhhhhh! I had psyched myself up for nothing!

As the voice message played, I had to make a quick decision whether to leave a message or just wait and call back later. Going through the "psyching up" process again was unappealing, so I opted for leaving a message asking him to call me back. Amazingly, he did.

When he asked to speak to me, I instantly knew who he was. The familiarity of his voice gave me a sense of comfort and relief. It was like I was in one of my dreams, madly looking for him, but now here he was, his voice signaling that my tormenting search had finally come to an end. I knew I had done the right thing.

We spent some time catching up on things like careers, children, and marriage. His tone was pleasant and void of anger or reservation. I had gotten past making the call, now I had to find the nerve to bring up the abortion. A pause in the conversation opened the door, so I walked right in. "I wanted to let you know I am now part of a post-abortion support group," I said casually. He then asked what the group was for. "Well, the abortion hurt me in a lot of ways, many of which I didn't know about until recently, so I joined to get help." I described my recurring dreams and then asked him if he remembered us ever talking about the baby or the abortion after it was done. He said we hadn't talked about it. Even though I had already arrived at the same conclusion, it still amazed me that we had never talked.

Well, why put it off any longer? I could tell he was ready, and I was ready, so we began the discussion that would hopefully bring closure to this aspect of the abortion. He told me he thought about the baby often. He regretted not having the baby, and he also shared that he felt guilty for not doing more to keep the baby.

I closed my eyes and sighed. He *was* hurt, and once again my heart ached for him. I felt a twinge of guilt that I was finally getting help, but he wasn't.

I briefly shared with him some of the emotional pain I had experienced, and then we reminisced about events surrounding the pregnancy. He recalled things that had escaped my memory. For instance, he reminded me that his mother offered to take the baby. I vaguely recalled that, but some of the details were still lodged in the anesthesia-induced fog in which I had lived throughout the whole ordeal.

I am reminded of when my son had surgery on the enlarged turbinates in his nose that impaired his breathing. In the recovery room after the surgery, we talked, but because he was still under the influence of the anesthesia, the next day, he had only a vague recollection of what either of us had said. I could relate.

When the conversation ended, I hung up the phone with a sense of completion. A gaping wound had just been stitched closed. One down, and who knows how many more to go?

chapter 8

He Turned My Mourning
into Joy

Throughout the years, my husband must have grown weary of me asking, "Do I look angry? His usual response was, "No." Then, my standard reply was, "Are you sure?"

I could not be convinced. When looking at myself in photographs taken without the premeditated "cheese" smile, my face, in its natural unsmiling state looked angry. Catching my reflection spontaneously in mirrors or glass panes confirmed it. I looked angry, but I didn't feel angry. Even my children sensed it.

While my family and I were eating dinner one day, I responded to something my oldest two children, who at the time were about eight and nine years old, said. I did not consider myself angry, but my son asked, "Why are you mad all the time?" He then said, "I don't want to have kids because kids make you mad."

His errant conclusion formed an invisible hand that struck me in the face. As I sat there motionless recovering from the sting of his words, feelings of failure filled my conscience. I had failed my kids. I had failed to demonstrate how much I loved them, how much of a blessing they were to me, and how fortunate I was to have them in my life. I failed to communicate to them the blessedness and privilege of having children.

I had been hit many times before by words that left me wounded; however, this slap was different. It was a wakeup call. Instead of wallowing in guilt and failure, I decided to step back and take a hard look at my actions and reactions. I had to see what Justin saw, and it was not pretty.

Through the process of self-examination, I discovered I had a serious "attitude." A seriously bad attitude. I was short-tempered with my husband and children; it took very little to annoy and agitate me. Yelling was a normal part of my interaction with my family.

In a study on managing conflict sponsored by my church, I learned that sarcasm is a manifestation of anger. As I listened to myself respond to my family, and as I listened to my thoughts in response to what others said or did (of course, I would never speak those thoughts aloud), sarcasm dripped from my words.

Unresolved anger develops into bitterness and Hebrews 12:15 describes bitterness as a *root*. Roots generally remain hidden underground, out of sight, but their fruit eventually breaks through the surface. I could not discern the feelings of anger because the root was hiding underground, but the wake up call forced me to take a close look at my behavior - the fruit - and it became apparent that not only did I look angry, but I was angry.

Hebrews 12:15 goes on to say that the root of bitterness will trouble us and thereby defile many. Justin's words at the table that day exposed the fact his beliefs about children had been defiled as a result of the root of bitterness embedded in me.

The next step was to determine the source of my anger. Now that I knew how it was manifesting, I controlled it as best I could with the help of the Holy Spirit, but it wasn't until four years later when the abortion issue came to a head that the actual root of the anger was exposed.

Rooting Out Anger

While working on the third lesson during the week prior to the group meeting, I was asked to describe my feelings before, during and after the abortion procedure, either physical or emotional. This is what I wrote:

" . . . *When I think of sitting in that recovery room, I get angry. I was also ashamed and embarrassed. . .I'll never forget when I got home, my dad was waiting at the door and when I came in, he hugged and hugged me. He was crying. He never said a word. Then I just went in my room and lay down. That was it. That was all that was said and all that was done. Makes me so ANGRY. My mom was there, my sister was there, but I don't recall any hugs . . .*"

I can't remember my emotional state when I responded to this question, but I noticed my handwriting changed when I wrote, "That was it. That was all that was said and all that was done. Makes me so ANGRY." It became messy, and the writing actually looked angry. My penmanship on subsequent questions returned to normal.

The next session dealt with anger. One of the questions in the book asked if there was anything about the abortion that I was or am still angry about. I wrote:

"Yes, 1) that I didn't have an option and I was robbed and violated, 2) no one helped me deal with it and 3) that they put me in that ridiculous recovery room."

At the time I answered this question in the book, I again do not recall any significant anger surfacing. However, it was a different story when the group met that week to discuss this lesson. When it was my turn to share my response to this question with the group, tears began rolling as I shared part one. Then, as I shared my experience in the recovery room, I cried harder and my voice got louder. Anger was rising. "It was so ridiculous and stupid to have us just sitting there looking at each other!" I angrily cried.

Then I moved on to describe the anger related to receiving no help in dealing with the abortion. The focus turned to my mother. "Afterward neither my mother nor my sister, who are women for Pete's sake, they didn't hug me or comfort me or anything! My father, a man, was the one who hugged me! They didn't do anything! No one said anything to me afterward! No one helped me! When it was over, that was it! My mom said nothing to me about it, ever! I was a kid! I didn't know how to deal with that!" The root of anger and bitterness was in full manifestation at this point. I was sitting on the edge of the sofa, yelling, my body shaking, and rivers of tears flowing down my cheeks.

When the outburst ended, my body still wracked with sobs, I came to myself and instantly became self-consciousness. I wondered what the other women were thinking about this forceful, emotional outburst. As I glanced around the room, I saw that every one of them was crying. Pat, the assistant facilitator who sat next to me, wrapped me in her arms and held me. They were "feeling" me, and it was a great comfort.

I had never realized how angry I had been with my mother, my sister, and the recovery room experience. The anger with my mom was not related to her decision to abort the baby because I always understood why she made that decision, but I was angry that she did not show me any kind of compassion or comfort and never did anything to help me through the trauma of that experience. As a child, I needed that from her. This was the unknown button that was pushed in the conversation weeks before when I told her about the group.

Finally giving vent to this suppressed anger, of which I was unaware, was healing in itself. The pressure in my chest was being released. Although drained, I felt lighter. It was obvious that I would have to release those with whom I was angry through forgiveness. Because healing was my goal, I willingly forgave.

Later that evening after returning home, I picked up my two-year-old son, Caleb, and coddled him on my lap. As he laid back on my chest, pain shot through the area on my chest under his head. I quickly sat him up, pulled out the top of my shirt by the collar and looked for the source of the pain, but nothing was visible.

As I undressed to take a shower the next morning, I glanced in the mirror, and a huge spot on my chest caught my eye; it was an enormous bruise. *Where did that come from?* In trying to figure it out, my mind wandered back to the group session the night before. I watched the replay of my angry outburst, and noticed something. At one of the times when I said "me," I simultaneously hit my chest with a balled-up fist. Because I was so enraged, I did not realize the force of that blow.

The image of the bruise on my chest paralleled the black rectangle I drew on my chest in the group's first session when Susan asked us to draw our pain. Then the Lord revealed to me that the icky heaviness I felt sitting my chest for years that began to surface when I watched the commercial, "Fifteen and Pregnant" was grief and anger. The spot where I hit myself is exactly where they sat. The bruise marked the spot and became a symbol that let me know that I would no longer feel that black, heavy sensation in my chest anymore. It had finally been released and I was free!

The bruise remained for almost two weeks, and each time I looked at it, even though it hurt like heck, I got happy. It reminded me of my freedom, and I knew that soon it would be gone, never to return, just like the bitter root of anger and grief that had weighed me down for over 20 years.

My Baby Has a Name

When the group began, Susan explained that there would be a memorial service in the eighth week. At each subsequent meeting she'd tell us a little a more about the service. As Mary had told me on the phone before the group began, Susan said we could name our babies if we desired, and their names would be used in the memorial service. She asked if we had a sense of our babies' gender, and of course, I did - he was a boy - and I was excited about naming him.

The names of my father, Herman, and my brother, Jeffery, who died of at the age 35, headed my list of possible names for my son. I only considered Herman because I wanted to name him after my father; otherwise, I am pretty sure it would have not made the list. Because I was single at the time of my pregnancy, his last name would be Blumenkrantz, but I couldn't settle on Jeffery Herman or Herman Jeffery. I really wanted to name him Herman Jeffery, but I didn't think I could actually give a child Herman as a first name.

I talked the names over with my husband, and as I did, a nagging voice developed in the back of my head saying, "You should be making this decision with the baby's daddy. It is *his* baby. He should have a part in deciding the name." I ignored it at first, but then I reluctantly came into agreement with it. He should be included in the naming process. He obviously thinks about our baby, and when he does, he should have a name, an identity, to relate to him.

It was easier to call him this time, and we had a great conversation. I told him about the upcoming memorial service and the importance of naming the baby and giving him an identity. I then expressed my desire for us to name the baby together. He was surprised, but he agreed. Although I had picked out names, I did not want to push them on him, so I asked if he had any names he preferred. There was a pause for a few seconds. Then he recommended we name him after my dad. I was floored. Out of the millions of names he could have picked, he chose the name I was considering. Wow.

I told him I wanted Herman, too, but wasn't sure if our baby would appreciate being called by that name. At the memory of the jesting my last name evoked, I could not bring myself to give my baby a name that could have made him a target for teasing. Even my dad used the name Jack instead of Herman.

No other name came to his mind, so I asked if our son's name could be Jeffery, my brother's name, and his middle name Herman. He consented.

So it was done. Our baby's name is Jeffery Herman Blumenkrantz.

Lightening the Load of Depression

Depression was an emotion with which I was all too familiar; it had been my constant companion from the time I aborted. I'll delve into this more later, but one of the chapters in the post-abortive Bible study book dealt with depression, and through it, the Lord revealed one of the "feeders" contributing to the load of depression weighing me down.

While working through the chapter at home, one of the passages of Scripture I read was Numbers 11. Here, Moses, the leader of the children of Israel, was unhappy because his followers were once again complaining and crying. On their journey through the wilderness, God had supernaturally supplied them with food from heaven - manna - but they were dissatisfied and longed for meat and the food they ate while in bondage in Egypt. Moses was then at his wits end because it seemed nothing he or God did ever satisfied the people. In his troubled state, he asked the Lord:

> Why have you brought this trouble on your servant? What have I done to displease you that you put the burden of all these people on me? Did I conceive all these people? Did I give them birth? Why do you tell me to carry them in my arms, as a nurse carries an infant, to the land you promised on oath to their fore-fathers? Where can I get meat for all these people? They keep wailing to me, 'Give us meat to eat!' I cannot carry all these people by myself; the burden is too heavy for me. (NIV)

Moses described his responsibility as a leader of this nation of people as a burden, a load he had to carry all alone; and it was too heavy for him. In his state of anguish and despair, he presented to the Lord his solution for escaping the weight he felt he could no longer bear. In Numbers 11:15 he says:

> If this is how you are going to treat me, put me to death right now - if I have found favor in your eyes - and do not let me face my own ruin. (NIV)

When God initially called Moses to deliver the children of Israel from Egypt, he struggled with accepting the call because of inadequacy issues. Now, the weight of the people and their continued discontentment made Moses feel even more inadequate, like a failure, and the only way of escape Moses saw was death. Although he would not take his own life, he asked God to favor him by killing him.

I was certain I had read this passage of scripture before, but now a new light of revelation was brightening my understanding of what Moses was experiencing. What was even more illuminating was God's response to Moses. He didn't berate him for his feelings of inadequacy or his death wish; neither did He try to encourage Moses to go on and be the leader He knew he could be. God's reply is given in Numbers 11:16:

> The Lord said to Moses: "Bring me seventy of Israel's elders who are known to you as leaders and officials among the people. Have them come to the Tent of Meeting, that they may stand there with you. I will come down and speak with you there, and I will take of the Spirit that is on you and put the Spirit on them. They will help you carry the burden of the people so that you will not have to carry it alone. (NIV)

I sat in awe as the light dawned on the significant implication of God's response to Moses. The bottom line is that it took seventy other people to help Moses carry the load he had been trying to carry alone. *Seventy!* That is a lot of people! No wonder Moses wanted to die - it was way too heavy.

Once I grasped this understanding, the Holy Spirit spoke to me and said I had been depressed and suicidal for so many years because I had been carrying the weight of the abortion and the loss of my child alone, and it was too much. One of the reasons I had carried that burden alone is because, unfortunately, I was unaware the emotional damage was linked to the abortion and the loss. I had not known until recently what had weighed me down like baggage loaded on a pack mule was abortion's aftermath.

Thanks be to God, that when the connection was finally made, He had prepared Pregnancy Counseling Center to help me once and for all deal with the heavy, burdensome weights like anger, grief, shame, and failure that had oppressed and depressed me almost to the point of suicide on numerous occasions. God was using the group leaders and the other women in the Bible study to help me just like he used the seventy elders to help lighten Moses' load. I did not have to carry it alone. My soul flooded with gratitude and relief. The load grew lighter as each week of the Bible study passed.

In looking at Moses' dilemma in Numbers 11, it became apparent to me that God knew all along that Moses could not handle the leadership of the nation of Israel alone. Thus, I asked Him why He did not just give Moses the other leaders to help him in the first place. The Lord showed me that Moses needed to know he could not handle it alone. When he got to that place, then he would gladly receive and appreciate the help.

This is exactly what happened to me. The Pregnancy Counseling Center had been in existence long before I found them in the paper. But it was not until I realized and admitted that I could not handle the issues resulting from the abortion alone, that God led me to them, and I willingly followed His lead. I was reared to be independent, and independent I was, so when problems arose in my life, I typically did not run to others for help. Even when others offered help, it was difficult to receive. With this situation, however, as with Moses', help is what enabled me to live.

Sad to say, there are many other women who have aborted and are carrying the burden of their abortions and the resulting emotional baggage alone. Shame compels them to keep it undercover. At times however, shame disguises itself as, "It's my business and no one else's. It was my personal decision and no one else needs to know." The need to feel strong and independent tells some they can handle it, they don't need help. Thus, women are trying to carry the abortion alone, yet are buckling under its weight. Some, even as Moses and I did, feel death is the only escape. My hope is that through my testimony, post-abortive women will realize there are people who desire to help bear their load and set them free from abortion's burdensome aftermath.

Jeffery in My Arms at Last

During one of our group sessions, Susan explained that we would be receiving a "doll" for each aborted baby to use as a tool in the grieving process. She then picked up a bag from which the "dolls" emerged. Each doll was made from a piece of cloth that was stuffed with a cottony material for the head, and a ribbon tied just under the head - a pink ribbon if the doll represented a girl, and a blue ribbon if the doll represented a boy. The rest of the cloth was left hanging free. In subsequent Bible study groups, women said the dolls looked like ghosts. I realized that was true once I heard it said, but when Susan handed me my doll with the little blue ribbon around its neck, its symbolism made a greater impact on me than its actual physical appearance. My breath caught in my chest as I held in my hands a tangible representation of my baby.

I was caught totally off guard. Susan had given no advance notice, or better yet, warning, that this would be part of the process, and the jury is still out on whether that was good or not. Tears began to well up in my eyes as I ever so gently held my "baby boy." I struggled to hold myself together as Susan continued giving instructions on what to do with the dolls. She stressed that the dolls were not meant to take the place of our babies, but they were to serve as tools to work through our grief issues. She informed us that we could do with them whatever we felt the need to do. Some women, she said, put the dolls away and never look at them again. Some hold them and talk with them. Some sleep with them. Some set them where they can see them, but never interact with them. It was totally up to us how we handled them. She told us that when we dedicated our babies during the memorial service, we would place them on the altar and leave them there, signifying we were committing them to God's care until we saw them again in heaven.

I kept the doll on the stand beside my bed where I could see it. Occasionally, I would pick it up, and draw it close as it somewhat soothed the aching in my arms for the child I never held. I would cry, tell Jeffery how much I loved him, and how sorry I was his life ended so soon. I stroked its head and straightened its ribbon. A couple of nights, I laid the doll in the bed between my husband and me where each of my four living children had spent many nights.

The Memorial Service

Although I was definitely freer than I had been in the past couple of decades, I anticipated the memorial service with conflicting emotions. I looked forward to the closure for the loss of my child, but I dreaded the emotional turmoil it would invoke. Death and funerals had always been extremely difficult for me. When my father passed, I begged my mom to excuse me from his funeral; it promised to be too overwhelming. She, however, said I needed to go to have closure. She was right. Though difficult, the funeral was not as bad as I had expected because of the support of so many family and friends, and their pleasant memories of my dad.

This would be different, though. The memorial service would not be attended by scores of family and friends who would lend their support and fond memories. There were no fond memories. The only memories of his short life were shrouded in pain. I knew for a certainty, however, I needed closure. I needed to call him by his name, to formally give him an identity and dedicate him to God. I knew I had to move on.

Susan asked us to prepare a special dedication for our baby, which we would present during the memorial service. She said we could write a letter to our baby and read it, or we could write a poem or do something artsy-craftsy. Because I love music so much, I decided to write a song for my son. The lyrics and melody flowed out of my heart. Although I love music, I am not a singer. Even if I could sing, however, I would not have been able to sing this particular song without breaking down somewhere close to the beginning. My husband picked up the melody on the piano and played it, but I did not want him to sing it. I thought it would be best for a female voice to carry the words from my heart to the heart of my child, so I asked my best friend, Melodie, a gifted psalmist, to learn and sing it. She agreed. Because the Bible study is confidential, all members of the group had to give their consent to those we wanted to invite to the service, and thankfully, everyone agreed my friend could come and sing.

The service took place in a small Presbyterian church. As I entered the sanctuary shortly before it was scheduled to begin, tears automatically fell from my eyes. My husband, Melodie and I took our seats on the front row. As I looked around the sanctuary, my tear-filled eyes fell on the minister who would be conducting the service, Pastor Mark. I had never seen him before, but Susan had assured us he was a Spirit-led man of God with great compassion for post-abortive women. He was Caucasian and looked to be in his mid-forties. I noticed that he kept blowing his nose. I wondered if maybe he had a cold. The longer I looked at him, however, I realized he was crying. Not only were I and the other women in the group crying, but he was crying also. I was deeply touched by his ability to "feel" us and our pain.

Susan opened the service with words of thanks to our visitors for their support and words of encouragement for the Bible study participants. Next, a woman with a sweet anointing sang songs of God's forgiveness and healing as she strummed her acoustic guitar. All we could do was cry, cry and cry. Tears of sadness and tears of healing.

Afterward, Susan called us up one by one to receive prayer and to dedicate our babies to the Lord. After she and Pastor Mark prayed a Spirit-led prayer for me, I took my place at the altar to dedicate Jeffery. I introduced Melodie and my husband who would sing and play the dedication song. As they did, we all continued crying. The lyrics to the song are:

Verse 1:

I was so young when you came along
I didn't have a clue what was going on
How precious your life was then
Or how hard mine would be
Once you were gone

Chorus:

I love you, my son
Though your life was short
And had barely begun
I love you, my son
But we'll see one another in a better place
Where there is no pain, shame or disgrace
I love you, my son. I love you, my son.

Verse 2:

Now my arms long to hold you
My eyes long to see you
My ears long to hear you say, Mom
But there's comfort in knowing you're with the Lord
And He's keeping you safe in His arms

Chorus:

Your brothers and sisters, you and me

Will live with God together, eternally
I love you, my son. I love you, my son.

I said, "I love you" to my son and committed him to the Lord as I laid the doll on the altar.

When the service ended, we fellowshipped over refreshments provided by a loving group of volunteers from another church. The repast was an effective way to help us transition from the emotionally-charged service to leaving somewhat emotionally intact. As my husband drove us home, I laid my head back on the headrest and closed my eyes, tired right down to the core, but certain my time of mourning was coming to an end.

Our last Bible study was the next week, and it was hard saying good-bye to Susan and Pat. They and Pastor Mark had been instrumental in bringing freedom to my soul. I still have the utmost respect and love for them, and I am continually thankful to God for their compassion and willingness to get in the trenches and cry with us and fight with us and for us.

A few days later during my personal devotion, I began to read the Psalms of David. I love the book of Psalms. I love how David expressed his admiration and praise to God. Sometimes when I just want to give God praise, I read aloud what David has written. On this particular day, I began to read Psalm 30 aloud, not realizing beforehand how much David's words paralleled what I had experienced in the preceding days, weeks and months. It says,

"I will extol thee, O Lord; for thou hast lifted me up, and has not made my foes to rejoice over me. O Lord my God, I cried unto thee, and thou hast healed me." (KJV)

This was my testimony! I cried to the Lord, and he healed me! Excitement and joy began to bubble up in my soul as I continued to read aloud.

"O Lord, thou hast brought up my soul from the grave: thou has kept me alive, that I should not go down to the pit."

I could hardly stand it! God had brought up my soul from the grave. I had been dying on the inside, and yearning to die on the outside, but He kept me alive. God kept me alive!

"Sing unto the Lord, O ye saints of his, and give thanks at the remembrance of his holiness. For his anger endureth but a moment; in his favor is life: weeping may endure for a night, but joy cometh in the morning."

Over twenty years of night and weeping had ended for me. This was my morning and joy belonged to me! I fell on my knees and choked on my sobs as I continued to read.

"And in my prosperity I said, I shall never be moved. Lord, by thy favor thou has made my mountain to stand strong; thou didst hide thy face, and I was troubled. I cried to thee, O Lord; and unto the Lord I made supplication. What profit is there in my blood, when I go down to the pit? Shall the dust praise thee? Shall it declare thy truth?"

It became clearer than ever before that the Lord valued my life. Dying would not profit Him at all. He kept me alive to praise Him and to declare his truth.

"Hear, O Lord, and have mercy upon me: Lord, be thou my helper. Thou hast turned for me my mourning into dancing: thou hast put off my sackcloth, and girded me with gladness; to the end that my glory may sing praise to thee, and not be silent. O Lord my God, I will give thanks unto thee forever."

Here, once again, David so perfectly expressed what I felt deep in my heart about the healing and restoration God had wrought in my life. He had turned my mourning into dancing. He had removed my mourning attire, and adorned me with gladness. I then knew there was no way I could keep silent about what I had experienced, regardless of how personal and controversial it was. I made the decision that I would declare the truth about abortion as God opened the doors, so that others would understand its destruction, and come to know the loving God that awaits the invitation to forgive, heal and restore. This is why I did not die. This is why He had kept me alive when I sometimes longed for Him to take me away. He knew my morning was coming. And He knew I would not keep silent.

The tears that fell from my eyes that day were not the familiar tears of sorrow or pain, but of joy, gladness and gratitude. Jesus had set me free, and my mandate had commenced. My mind was made up that I would do all I possibly could to deliver women from the agonizing pain of abortion, either by prevention or by ministering post-abortion healing.

chapter 9

It Takes a Thief

As recorded in John 10:10, Jesus said, "The thief cometh not, but for to steal, and to kill, and to destroy . . ." (KJV)." This passage of Scripture refers to Satan, and in light of it, we understand his sole intention - to steal, kill and destroy. Abortion is a highly successful method of achieving this goal. Not only is a baby's life destroyed, but also in the process of aborting, a woman is robbed of precious possessions which under gird her sense of fulfillment and contentment in being uniquely woman.

Self-worth is stolen, and replaced with shame and condemnation. Peace is stolen and replaced with a distressing void. Trust is stolen and replaced with doubt, fear and distrust. Joy is stolen and replaced with depression. A sense of calm is stolen and replaced with anger. Security is stolen and replaced with violation. And the list goes on. Once these things have been snatched away, Satan's plan of destruction becomes easier to accomplish.

For twenty-two years, I was robbed. The revelation of the extent to which I had been robbed dawned on me recently. While sitting in my office working, John 10:10 suddenly popped into my mind. Although there is more to this Scripture, I thoughtfully mulled over the fact that Satan seeks only to steal, kill and destroy.

Then, as if I was seated in a movie theater, my life began to play on the screen of my mind. I watched as the four main goals I had set for myself while in junior high school became reality in their prioritized order. I saw myself accomplish my first goal of getting married in July of 1983. The fulfillment of my second goal materialized when I became pregnant with my first-born son in June, 1984. I watched as I walked (or more appropriately, waddled) down the commencement aisle to receive my B.B.A. in accounting in December, 1984, my third goal, while six months pregnant. I saw myself hired as an accountant - my first job that paid "real" money.

By the time I was 26, I had attained my four main goals. What an accomplishment! As this mental biography played in my mind, I should have experienced an awesome sense of satisfaction and fulfillment, but I didn't. My accomplishments were tainted as I watched myself struggle internally over the years with various fears, hatred, self-hatred, depression, suicide, anger, guilt, and shame. I watched my relationships with my husband and children suffer due to my own emotional distress. Although I had embraced my dream, I was unable to completely enjoy its benefits. I saw the prime of my life stolen from me. I saw the relationship for which I had longed with my children snatched away.

As this revelation unfolded before me, initially, I was saddened. Then I grew indignant. How dare Satan do this! Thank God for the rest of John 10:10, which I will discuss in further detail later. At this point, however, I want to offer a closer look at the devastating effects of my abortion which Satan used to rob me and devised to ultimately destroy me.

Before I begin, however, please be aware that abortion is not just a physical act, but is the result of what is called "spiritual warfare." The spirit realm, where God and his holy angels abide, is also inhabited by demons, or fallen angels. Many people don't believe in God, and even more don't believe in Satan or demons. But whether one believes or not, they exist. There is a constant battle raging in the spirit realm that we, as humans, cannot see with our physical eyes, but in which we are actively involved. In fact, much of the warfare revolves around us.

"Deliverance" is one means of engaging in spiritual warfare, and is basically the ministry of casting out demons. God gives His people the authority and power to cast them out of people whom they have bound (Mark 16:17). A teaching on spiritual warfare and deliverance is a vast undertaking, which I am well able to handle, but unfortunately is beyond the scope of this book. There are, however, numerous resources available on this topic, some of which can be found on a website noted at the end of this book.

Much of what I am about to address involves spiritual warfare - deliverance, in particular.

The Weighty Baggage

My most vivid memory some time after the abortion is standing at the kitchen sink in my mother's house holding a knife to my wrist. A humongous, oppressive weight with an unknown origin had settled on me, and at that point, carrying it around had become unbearable. Because I did not know what it was or from whence it came, the only means of escaping its oppressive, downward force was to take my life. As I stared at the knife lying flat on the inside of my wrist, I wondered how it would feel sliding across my skin hard enough to sever the green veins visible through my seemingly transparent skin.

It did not take long to arrive at a conclusion: *That will hurt.* Almost immediately, a strong aversion to self-inflicted pain prevailed over the desire to end it all. Thoroughly disgusted with myself, I put the knife down, and carried on as miserable as ever.

Externally, I appeared to be doing well. I excelled in high school and eventually graduated second in my class. I was a cheerleader, class secretary, and was even voted homecoming queen. Aside from the regular drama brought on by the jealous and ignorant, one would think my life was great. Good home training on "moving on," coupled with the numbness masking my pain's root, enabled me to outwardly do well despite the inner turmoil. Well, that is, except for the fact that not a single day passed that I didn't cry. Sometimes I knew why I cried, other times I did not.

Not long after my cowardly retreat from suicide, I developed a constant upset stomach. After several complaints about it, my mom took me to the doctor (yes, the same doctor that confirmed my pregnancy), but he could find no cause. He suggested to her some sort of emotional stress as the root. Their eyes simultaneously settled on me while they waited for me to confirm or dissent. I merely lowered my head, shrugged my shoulders and mumbled, "I don't know." As feeble as it sounded, this was the absolute truth. I had no idea what was going on with me. I felt trapped in a dense fog that kept me totally blinded to the source of the anxiety and burden weighing me down.

After a year or so, I adjusted to life with the heaviness and the crying. The additional baggage and the weeping had become a part of me, and just like someone with a permanent physical handicap, I learned to function despite it. Regardless of how unsettling it was at times, this was now me. These things had woven themselves into the fabric of my identity. To friends and family, I was known as a "crier." As I stated before, I am and have always been emotional, as well as sensitive, and I believe this is part of my true self that God created for what He has purposed me to do. However, the crying that was now manifesting was far beyond the real me, only I wasn't aware of it.

My usual response to the question, "How are you?" became "Tired." I admired and sometimes even envied high-energy women because I forever felt like I was dragging. Never enough energy. Carrying around baggage all day everyday will have that effect on you.

The Addiction

Having an abortion and losing a parent within a nine-month period is quite a heavy emotional load for a 15-year-old to handle alone. I had packed the abortion-related trauma in my emotional baggage and stored the bags in my invisible closet, but other mechanisms for coping with this load unconsciously kicked in.

Foremost, I clung to my boyfriend as never before. The emotional and physical affection we shared helped soothe my hurting soul. He wasn't allowed to visit me at home for a few months after the abortion, but I spent as much time with him as possible at school, during and after school hours. Whenever we were apart, my whole being ached to be with him. I have no doubt some would mistakenly label this vehement desire as "love." While it sounds sweetly romantic, the truth is, he was a pain killer to which I was addicted, and as with any addict, I couldn't get enough of him.

While painkillers are helpful in managing pain, their primary disadvantage is they don't provide a cure for its cause; they mask it. Once their effectiveness has lapsed, the pain returns. Thus, another one is needed; and the cycle continues, leading many to addiction. This is how I became addicted to relationships, not with just my boyfriend, but with men in general. It began with the ache of rejection and became severe after the abortion. After one relationship ended, I had to move on to the next. Sometimes, though not often, I had to double the dose and maintain two relationships at the same time.

I reiterate, at the time, I did not understand the driving force behind my neediness of and clinginess in relationships. It felt like the natural thing to do and developed into another trait composing my ever-evolving false identity.

Alcohol became another painkiller. My family had always enjoyed drinking, and casually shared a little here and there with me throughout my childhood. Like my family, I also enjoyed drinking. I liked the taste of alcohol, and I liked the silly, giddy feeling resulting from a few sips. The bar in our basement provided a fairly accessible supply. In reality, I did not drink excessively everyday, but when the weights got especially heavy, triggered by the ignorant and jealous at school, or trouble with my boyfriend, or, as in most cases, by inexplicable unseen influences, I'd overindulge.

Every now and then, I'd also use my other pain numbing medication - sleep. Because I was very active in high school, I wasn't able to use it as much. But when nothing else was available, this one worked just fine.

Basically, I was addicted to painkillers. Not your usual painkillers like Vicadin or other narcotics, but emotional painkillers. I had places to go, people to see, things to do, so it became imperative to use whatever was available to lighten my load and ease the pain. I was just like an injured boxer or football player who wants to stay in the fight or the game, and will resort to whatever measures it takes to get back in it.

Other post-abortive women have addictions that help them escape their reality. They may be the same as mine, but there are many others. Some throw themselves into school or their careers, while others strive to become "supermom." They are addicted to overachievement; the busyness distracts from the pain, and the success helps them feel better about themselves.

If a woman aborted because of her career, then the success also makes her feel justified for aborting, thus numbing the pain. Overachieving as "supermom" also helps the pain in a couple of ways: one, it is used to dull the painful, nagging voice of condemnation which says, "You're a bad mother because you killed your baby;" and two, it is used to provide compensation to a living child(ren) for what an aborted child lost.

The fact of the matter is, until the cause of the pain is dealt with, the pain will never completely go away. Relationships or achievements or temporary highs from drugs or whatever emotional pain killer is abused cannot bring true healing to the soul who has aborted. Only God can do that.

The Lord Saved Me

After graduating from high school, I started college, and it was there in my freshman year, that I truly made Jesus my Lord. Young people who loved the Lord surrounded me, and their fire and passion set me ablaze.

One of the first things after salvation the Lord dealt with me about was the abortion. Having discussed it with no one, but by the conviction of the Holy Spirit only, I recognized that this act was not only wrong, but it was indeed a sin. It was murder, so I asked God to forgive me. I asked in faith, and I believed whole-heartedly He had forgiven me and the blood of Jesus had washed the sin away. Once again, I thought it was over; but not so.

The Miscarriage

Having children ranked number two on my life-goals list right under getting married. I didn't just want to have children; I wanted to have *lots* of children. My grandmother, after whom I am named and who I admired dearly, had eleven children and I wanted to be like her. Well, almost - I'd be satisfied with ten.

Although my husband and I had not planned to have children right away, within the first year of marriage, I was pregnant with our first baby. Because of a lack of funds and health insurance, I had to take the pregnancy test at a local clinic where they were administered for free. When I called about taking the test, the clinic's receptionist told me my period had to be at least two weeks late before taking the test.

My continued lack of diligence in keeping track of my period resulted in me once again struggling to remember when I had my last one. After settling on a fairly reliable date, I performed the calculations to determine when I'd qualify to take the test. Because I had to drop off a first-morning-urine sample on the day of the test, I stopped by the clinic a few days before to pick up the empty cup.

My breasts were tender, but sometimes that happened when my cycle was about to start, so I didn't get my hopes up.

I dropped off the sample at the clinic on my way to work one Friday morning.

As the day wore on, I began to feel a slight sensation of cramping in my lower back. A couple of hours later, the cramps became more intense. I went to the bathroom to check whether anything was happening, and sure enough, my period had started. I felt some initial disappointment, but after a few minutes, I bounced back. Being pregnant would have been a dream-come-true, but since we weren't planning to have a baby this soon anyway, it was no big deal.

Soon after returning to my desk, the phone rang. Once the lady on the other end identified herself as a nurse at the clinic, I knew why she was calling. She was calling to say the test was negative, of course, because my period had started.

"Your test," she said, "was positive." *What?* "I'm sorry," I said. "Could you say that again; I didn't hear what you said." She repeated, "Your test was positive."

Wow! I'm pregnant?! Excitement swelled in me for a few seconds, until I suddenly remembered the bleeding and cramping. I informed the nurse, and she said that happens sometimes, but if it got worse to call them back. The fact that the blood was not an automatic sign of miscarriage allayed the fear and panic I felt beginning to mount.

I hung up the phone ecstatic, and I couldn't wait to tell my husband. The news of our first child had to be shared in person, though, so I'd have to contain myself until I got home. The longer I sat at work, however, the worse the cramps and the bleeding became. By the time I left later that afternoon, the cramps had reduced me to tears, and I was passing clots.

I called the clinic, and because it was late on a Friday, they told me they couldn't see me until Monday. I was tormented the entire weekend. In the back of my mind I knew I was miscarrying, but I could not accept it. I could not accept I was losing a baby.

On Monday, the doctor at the clinic examined me and gave me another test. He confirmed it; I had miscarried. It was unbelievable. Just unbelievable. If I had just waited one more day to take the test, I would have never known I was pregnant. I would have only assumed this was a particularly difficult period. All of my cycles were pretty painful and heavy, and I wouldn't have suspected anything unusual about this one if I hadn't gone to take the test.

I cried out to God, "Why did I have to find out I was pregnant? Why did it have to happen this way?" It seemed so unfair. Why couldn't the bleeding have started the day before the test? I would not have then taken the test. Hoping I was pregnant and then starting my period was one thing; but knowing I was pregnant, if only for a minute, and then miscarrying was something I lacked the emotional strength to handle.

Later that week, while cleaning out my pockets, I found a crumpled piece of paper. While smoothing it out with my hands, I discovered it was the receipt from the clinic for the exam that confirmed my miscarriage (unfortunately, the exam wasn't free). My eyes fell upon the two words handwritten on the diagnosis line. "Spontaneous abortion." This term was unfamiliar to me. My eyes locked on the word "abortion." *Abortion? I had another abortion?* It took a few seconds to pull my puzzled gaze from "abortion" to "spontaneous." A few more seconds passed, and then it clicked. *Oh, I get it! It's just another term for miscarriage.* Although pleased with myself for solving the puzzle and learning something new, I continued to stare at the words, still shocked by the terminology. Finally, I put it away. But I couldn't put the pain away.

I hurt. Real bad. All things considered, including the fact that I was very young at the time, only 23, and that we were not even trying to get pregnant, the depth of depression to which I sank was extreme. For three months, I cried endlessly. My strength was sapped, and performing my usual daily routine felt like a climb up Mount Everest. A devastating disappointment and sorrow shrouded me. My husband felt helpless in trying to comfort me; all he could do was pray.

Looking back on it, I now understand the sorrow, disappointment and grief seemingly sucking the life from me was not solely for the loss of my miscarried baby. This loss unknowingly pried open the locked closet and baggage in which the unresolved pain and grief from the loss of my aborted baby had been stored.

Three months after the miscarriage I believe God extended his mercy to me, and if not me, then certainly my husband, and I was pregnant again. Although we had not planned this pregnancy either, I was once again ecstatic. This good news helped stuff my abortion baggage back in the closet, though certainly did not rid me of it.

1 John 4:18 says "fear has torment," and although I did not miscarry this pregnancy, the fear of losing the baby relentlessly tormented me for the first three months. I bled a little every single day from the time I read the positive results of my home pregnancy test until three months later.

Two of my friends were also pregnant during this time, and a sickening jealousy rolled in me as I watched them enjoying their pregnancies while I suffered daily anxiety. All I ever wanted was to be pregnant and enjoy the process, but joy had been robbed from me. I wanted so much to bond with my growing baby, but the spirit of fear caused me to keep a safe distance, just in case the blood was a sign I would miscarry. I had been pregnant with two babies and had lost them both. Maybe because of the abortion, I would never birth a baby. (Satan isn't just a thief; he is also a liar. I not only birthed a baby, I birthed five.)

Relating to My Children

As I reflected on my relationship with my children, especially my oldest two, it was apparent the thief had robbed me of the joy that comes with motherhood.

During my childhood, I loved children, and I had plenty opportunities to express this love with younger cousins and my brother's children. I cared for my niece and nephew just as I imagined I would care for my own children one day. I was twelve years old when my first nephew was born, and my brother would often bring him to my mom's house for baby-sitting. When he was just an infant, my mom consented, after some begging, to let him sleep with me, so I could care for him during the night. He joined me in my twin bed, and when he'd awaken in the middle of the night, I'd give him his bottle. Afterward, I would lay him on my chest and gently rock him until he drifted soundly to sleep. I'd bathe him and his sister, wash their hair, dress and feed them, and change their diapers. It was great! I could hardly wait to have my own. A couple of years after the abortion, however, something horrible manifested.

My sister gave birth to a son about a year after I aborted. She lived with us in my mom's house, so I was able to spend quality time with him, and I enjoyed every minute. One day, when he was somewhere between one and two years old, while I carried him from my house to my grandmother's house across the street, he inconsolably cried and screamed. I was pretty used to children crying and screaming, but on this particular day, the noise of his cries struck a hidden chord. An instantaneous burst of anger surged from me and I began to shake him, and then hit him, all the while yelling for him to be quiet. Of course, he screamed louder, and when my tirade was over, I was shaking. I swooped him up from his seat on my grandmother's driveway, and carried him back to my house. Obviously, I couldn't deal with him right then, so I thought it'd be best to leave him with his mom.

After returning him to his mom, the familiar feelings of shame and condemnation made me bow my head and cry. I could not believe I treated him that way; he was just a baby. *What is my problem?* The answer never came.

I continued babysitting my nieces and nephews, and never again experienced an outburst or even a hint of anger like the explosion that day. That is until my first child, Justin, was born. Justin and I had issues bonding from the very beginning, as I mentioned before. Unfortunately, after he was born, it worsened. I loved my baby so much, and I wanted to be the best mom he could ever have, but it felt like all hell had been let loose to preclude such a thing from happening. He was a strong-willed child, and I was an angry mother - not a very good combination - and at the time, what I was angry about was anybody's guess.

My responses to his normal infant and toddler behavior were harsh. It is embarrassing and extremely difficult to admit, but at times, some of what my son endured could be labeled "abuse." The fact that my behavior was in such stark contrast to the intent of my heart, set me up for satanic attacks of suicide. Although it happened infrequently, one of my outbursts of either screaming, yanking, hitting or some combination of the three would send me spiraling down the slippery slope of "you're a bad mother," and landing me in the valley of "you don't deserve to live."

Please don't get me wrong. Justin and I had great times. He was my son and I wouldn't have traded him for anything. I never regretted having him, or any of my children for that fact, but we were definitely not experiencing a healthy mother/son relationship. When he began to talk, he called me "Lydia" and called his dad, "Mom." This cut me to the core, and his use of those names was a painful reminder that I and my relationship with him had fallen way short of my hopes and expectations. I am a realist, so I was not expecting a perfect, problem-free relationship with my children. But I knew beyond a shadow of a doubt, we were lingering on the far left side of normal. I, and my son, had been robbed.

Disappointment and condemnation remained my constant companions. I am so thankful, though, that Jesus said *He* would never leave me nor forsake me (Hebrews 13:5), and that He would be a friend that sticks closer than a brother (Proverbs 18:24). His companionship, rich with grace and mercy, overshadowed the disappointment and condemnation and gave me hope when hopelessness threatened to overtake me. He continually assured me everything would be all right.

When Justin was ten months old, I was pregnant, and once again, I was thrilled. There was no spotting in this pregnancy, but a fear of losing the baby still stealthily lurked, craftily corrupting my ability to bond with my developing daughter.

This pregnancy presented me another opportunity to fulfill my dream of having a happy, healthy relationship with my children. Christen was born, and we got off to a great start. Soon after her birth, however, I had got a bad case of the baby blues. I was warned this could happen, but the warning did not assist at all in pulling me out of it. My changing hormones put me on the familiar road to the valley of depression and once there, I met up with its long time inhabitants, "you're a bad mother," and "you deserve to die." *Why couldn't I be normal?* My friends who were starting their families appeared to wear motherhood well. *Why was I struggling?*

Soon after having Christen, Tim and I decided we were done having children. We both worked full-time and also bore a lot of responsibility in our church. This, combined with having two children under the age of two, wore us out; and of course, I was fully persuaded no other child should be subjected to my ineptness as a mother. My dream of having ten children was put out of its misery (not that my husband bought into it in the first place), and I convinced myself I could be very happy with two. I was only 25 then, and for some reason, I could not even imagine having another child. Generally, I am able to produce a mental picture of what I want or even might want in my mind before I receive it (you know, see it before I see it), but I could not muster up any kind of image of our family with more than two children. There was nothing there; so we decided to get my tubes tied.

This was a major decision and before making major, life-changing decisions, Tim and I seek counsel from our pastor. When we met with him and told him what we wanted to do, he advised against it. He did not think it was a wise decision.

Tim and I trust our pastor because we know he is a man of God who hears from God and sincerely loves us. Therefore, despite the certainty we felt about getting the procedure done, we followed his counsel and left my tubes just as they were. We did, however, get super serious about birth control. Our days of youthful carelessness were over and we faithfully exercised our right to choose protection.

Some eighteen years and three more kids later, our pastor still lightheartedly reminds us of his role in the size of our fairly large family.

Hatred of Children

My church sponsored its first workshop on the deliverance ministry. The minister leading this event was from Chicago, and he provided us a manual he had written on deliverance. In it, terms associated with deliverance were listed in alphabetical order, and next to each term was an explanation and related Bible scriptures.

This manual was used during the workshop, but because of time restraints, we were unable to work through it entirely. I strongly felt deliverance ministry was a significant part of my personal calling, and I wanted to be well-informed and skilled, so I took it to work to study on my breaks.

When the first break of the day rolled around, I picked up the manual and opened it to the first page. To my surprise, the first word in this alphabetical list of deliverance terms was "abortion." *What?* I thought to myself when I saw it. *What does abortion have to do with casting out demons?* Its explanation comprised two short paragraphs, but as I read the words, tears started flowing from my eyes; and by the last word of the last paragraph, I was choking back gut-wrenching sobs.

The revelation that abortion gave entrance to demons that could bind the mind, will, and emotions was surprising and very disturbing; yet, at the same time, it was comforting. It felt as if a missing piece in the understanding of my inner turmoil had clicked into place.

While trying to keep the volume of my cries low in my small office cubicle, I picked up the phone and called my pastor's wife. She was my good friend, and a spiritual giant. "What's the matter?" she said after I choked out my greeting. I told her about what I had read and that something related to it was manifesting through me right there in my office. I asked her if she would minister to me because I wanted to get free.

Before I called her, I had formulated a plan that consisted of me going to her home after work where she would then pray for me, but she had a different plan. She told me she would minister to me at our annual youth retreat two weeks away. *Two weeks! I couldn't wait two weeks!* "But they're manifesting now! I can't wait two weeks." I cried.

"Yes, you can" she said calmly. "Jesus gave you authority over those spirits, so go into the bathroom right now and bind them up. Tell them they have to stop."

"Okay," I said. If she said I could do it, then I could. I went in the bathroom and told the spirits, "I bind you in the name of Jesus. You will stop manifesting and when the first lady ministers to me at the retreat, you will come out." I felt my composure returning, but the revelation was still stunning. The abortion made me vulnerable to demonic oppression. Who knew? Right there in the bathroom stall, the light of that revelation produced a glimmer of hope that shone through the dark cloud of doom and gloom ever hovering over me. Maybe there were other forces influencing my behavior, and my true self was not an inadequate wife and mother. Maybe I was not doomed to carry this heavy load of guilt and shame. Maybe I really could be a good mother and wife.

Two weeks later, we made our way to the youth retreat, and true to her word, she prayed for me during the first altar call of the weekend. Because neither of us was aware abortion spirits existed until two weeks before, we were not certain with what spirits I had been bound, but she started with the spirits of abortion and murder.

Those spirits left as she ministered to me, but then the Holy Spirit gave her discernment of another spirit that had entered as a result of the abortion. Hatred of children. When she called the name of that spirit, it immediately began to cry out. I thought to myself, *I don't hate children.* Having been through deliverance training, though, I knew a person could be bound with spirits of which he or she was unaware - like the abortion and murder spirits. The fact that it was manifesting made its presence obvious, so I went with the flow. After much protesting, it left.

Once the deliverance was over, I felt different - my load felt a little lighter, especially in my mind. Praise filled my mouth, and I expressed to God over and over my appreciation of His mercy, grace, and love for me.

A few minutes later, I experienced a drastic change that left me awe-filled. Before the deliverance, it was impossible for me to mentally formulate a picture of my family with more than the two children I had. After the deliverance, however, I easily envisioned more children. It was an amazing feeling of freedom. My mind and attitude regarding children had been set free from a small, tightly enclosed space, and the Lord showed me Hatred of Children had been its walls.

As time went on, the Lord gave me greater clarity on how this spirit affects people. Its influence can range anywhere from subtle to blatant. Of course, its blatant influence can be seen in those who actually claim they hate children. A step below blatant can look like constant criticism or intolerance. With me, it had to take a more subtle approach because by the time I had aborted, my love for children was already a settled issue. "I hate children" is something I would never buy into, so it took another form.

I never saw this before, but the Lord showed me I sometimes became angry at my young children's behavior, many times age-appropriate, because the influence of this spirit made me believe they were really a burden. They just wanted to keep me from doing what I wanted and needed to do. If things didn't go as smoothly as *I* thought they could or should, like potty training or if they cried too much, or wanted, in my thinking, too much attention, I took it personally - they were doing these things just to annoy me or make my life miserable. I saw them as hindrances to my personal happiness.

When you think about it, this is exactly the influence behind many decisions to abort. We have other things we need to do and having a child would either keep us from doing them, make it more difficult or slow us down. We hear its influences telling us children are a financial burden, and we can't afford them. We hear they are a time burden, and we don't have time for them. We hear they are a hindrance to attaining real success. While these influences may be external, once they convince us to abort, the spirit then gains access to inhabit and control our emotions, minds, and wills, many times forcing us in directions opposite the true intent of our hearts.

This spirit, along with the spirit of murder is what caused me and many other mothers to cross the line between discipline and abuse. I believe because through it all, I sought the Lord God with all my heart, His Spirit kept me from crossing this line as far as others have.

The Hatred of Children also influences many to remain childless, and again this influence can range from subtle to blatant. One just has to listen to the reasons for having no children.

Because the enemy purposed to destroy me, though, his plan for me was to watch me fulfill my dream of having children, and then unleash this spirit which had remained pretty much dormant since the abortion (with the exception of the incident with my nephew) to wreak havoc in my relationship with my children. This in turn would feed my feelings of being a horrible mother, which in turn would feed "you're don't deserve to live" feelings. Ultimately, he wanted me to kill myself, and this was just one strategy to make this happen.

Thanks be to God, however, He also had a plan for me, which had nothing to do with me dying, and everything to do with me living and having abundant life, even in my family. God's plan is greater than Satan's any day, and He will watch over us to ensure His plan is fulfilled.

In Jeremiah 29:11, God says:

> For I know the plans I have for you, says the Lord, plans for welfare and not for evil, to give you a future and a hope. (NIV)

God's plan for me and for you is not evil. He wants to give us a hope and a future, regardless of how bad our situation looks. As I said before, we are in spiritual warfare, and the enemy of our souls is cunningly devising ways of destroying us. I am so glad that in Christ, we win. We may lose a few battles, but the war and the victory belong to those who have been washed in the blood of the Lamb.

Jesus had set me free from spirits of hatred of children, murder and abortion. Unfortunately, because of my bondage during the delicate first three and four years of my two oldest children's lives, their innocent souls were damaged. For years, I was tormented with guilt regarding this, yet I prayed earnestly that God would heal my children's spirits and souls. As usual, He came through. More about this later, though.

Fear and the Inability to Bond

After this deliverance, my relationship with my children improved considerably, but I sensed something still stood between us. It's as if the abortion's aftermath was an onion and layers were slowly being peeled back. Once one or two were gone, there was another to face.

One evening, I sat in my living room thinking about my children and how much I loved them. I began to sense there was something specific blocking me from fully giving myself to them and loving them like I knew I could. I did not get into a deep prayer; I just asked God while I sat there, "What is it? What is the block?" He immediately responded.

His voice was clear when he said, "You have a fear of losing of your children. Because you think you'll lose them, you will not allow yourself to fully bond with them. It's a means of protecting yourself from the pain of loss."

"Oh my God," I whispered. I had an inkling of this when I was pregnant with Justin, and an even slighter one when pregnant with Christen. However, I never recognized this once they were born. Another puzzle piece snapped into place.

Honestly, I don't know how I missed it. There were signs; the most glaring of which was my extreme overprotectiveness. I did not like them taking risks, climbing on things or being out of my sight for a minute. I was forever saying, "Come back," Get down," or "Don't touch that!" Their curiosity and sense of exploration had been stifled because of my fear.

After the Lord spoke to me, my mind went back to an incident that happened shortly before this particular evening. Justin and I were sitting on the floor and I told him to stop doing something - it wasn't something wrong, but something I thought was dangerous. He then innocently asked, "Mom, why are you so scared?" I instantly knew to what he was referring, and I just stared at him for a minute. My four-year-old son had discerned the fear in me.

Discernment is one of my strongest gifts, but I had not discerned this fear. I had reasoned that I was only trying to be a good mother by looking out for the well-being of my children. Justin's insight surprised me, but I didn't address it then.

Now it was becoming clearer. I was afraid of losing them. This is why I had been so overprotective. I thanked God for giving me this revelation; but while I was thankful, I was also sad. The importance of bonding with infants had been explained to me in a Child Psychology class I had in college, as well as in literature I read while pregnant. We had bonded to some extent, but far short of where we could have been. Fear was another thief that had robbed me of a close relationship with my young children. Interestingly, though, I was not totally delivered from this fear of losing my children until about four years later.

I had made a conscious effort to relax and give my children a little more freedom, but the fear began to manifest in another way. Vivid scenarios of them being kidnapped or dying in an accident would suddenly materialize in my mind. The entire episode would play out, and by its conclusion, I'd be sobbing.

My mother-in-law fell gravely ill in Alabama, and for about three weeks, Tim would often travel there to see her. When he'd leave, the subtle fear that rumbled under the surface when he was home would explode into a horrendous torment that kept me wide-eyed and panicky as I lay in bed at night. Fear the house would catch on fire, and I would be unable to save my children constantly plagued my mind. With Tim gone, I would be unable to protect them if the house caught on fire. The concern was never for me, just for my kids.

Unfortunately, Tim's mom died, and once he returned home, the fear became less intense, but it never left. Up to this point, I had not told anyone, not even Tim, with what I was struggling; I just kept it to myself, hoping it would go away. But eventually, I got to a point where I could not live with it any longer. Fear, no matter how strong or how subtle, is a thief, and for years, the torment of this fear had robbed me of peace. It had robbed me of sleep. It had robbed me of joy. It had robbed me of rest. This spirit of fear had to go! It was not of God because 2 Timothy 1:7 says: "For God hath not given us the spirit of fear; but of power, and of love, and of a sound mind." (KJV)

One thing is true about deliverance: in order to be free, you have to *desperately* want it, and I wanted it bad. I asked for prayer during altar call at my church. After the prayer, I felt relief for a while, but the same fear soon returned. At this point, I asked one of the women in ministry at my church to join my husband in ministering deliverance to me.

She came to my home, and while she and Tim prayed, the Lord gave her a word of knowledge about this spirit of fear. She said it was a fear of losing my children, and it had gained entrance through my abortion. She explained that because I was unable to protect the child I lost, I feared being unable to protect and subsequently losing my children.

When she said this, a scream resonated from the depths of my inner being. The Lord had exposed the root of the bondage, so now, the spirit had no choice but to leave and take its torment with it!

The truth had set me free, and I have not been tormented with this fear since.

In Psalm 34:4, David says, "I sought the Lord and he heard me, and delivered me from all

my fears." (KJV)

God is so good!

Sexual Issues

For the first year of marriage, I enjoyed intimacy and making love with my husband. The second year, the enjoyment decreased; by the third year, I could take it or leave it; and by the fifth year, I couldn't stand it. During our lovemaking, I sometimes had to battle the urge to scream or fight the overwhelming compulsion to place both my hands on his chest and push him off me. At other times, I got nauseous to the point of almost throwing up. My husband is a wonderful lover, so I did not understand what was happening. Once again, I cried out to God for help.

While waiting for an answer, I saw an advertisement for a book about ministering to women who had abortions. I ordered it, and it arrived on a day when our church had its midweek service. I quickly read through the book after dinner, and as I did, I felt something stirring inside me. My stomach felt as if it had butterflies flitting around, and I guessed these were other abortion-related spirits that had been stirred by the book.

Of course, when the invitation for altar prayer was given that night at church, I was the first one at the altar. A dear sister prayed for me, but I did not specify a prayer request because I wasn't sure what exactly had been roused. While praying, this sister suddenly said in an authoritative voice, "In the name of Jesus, I rebuke the spirit of uncleanness and command you to go!" After a few minutes of intense warfare, this spirit left.

I lay on my side on the floor feeling somewhat drained and a little embarrassed; then a new, unfamiliar feeling began to emerge. As I stood to walk back to my seat, tears of joy streamed from my eyes, and praise flowed from lips because I knew I was different - I was clean! This feeling of clean was the cleanest clean I ever felt. It was overwhelming! I never realized how dirty I was until I was made clean. It's like not realizing how gray an old white shirt has become until it is placed next to a bright, new shirt. I felt indescribably pure.

As the service continued, I knelt at my seat, crying and whispering praise to God for the awesome miracle wrought for me that night. His power, so amazing and absolute, delivered me and transformed me in an instant.

After arriving home, I tearfully recounted the events of my miracle to my husband. He sat quietly and listened as I feebly attempted to explain this newfound sensation of "clean." I gave up after realizing I had no words to describe it. At that point, he rose from his seat on the floor, sat at our old electric piano and begin to play and sing in his soothing, melodic timbre "Whiter than Snow."

I fell on my face on the floor, as, once again, Tim displayed his sensitivity to the Holy Spirit and my feelings by accurately articulating in song what I was unable to express in words. Yes, that's how I felt - whiter than snow. Washed and cleansed. As I lay there prostrate, the words of this prayerful melody flowing from my husband's lips felt like a waterfall flowing over my heart, soul and body, cleansing me even more. He sang:

> "Lord Jesus, I long to be perfectly whole,
> I want Thee forever to live in my soul.
> Break down every idol, cast out every foe–
> Now wash me and I shall be whiter than snow.
> Whiter than snow, yes, whiter than snow–
> Now wash me and I shall be whiter than snow"

The Lord had revealed in prayer that night that this spirit had come in through the abortion. I had been forgiven of the sin, but again, it had opened the door to an unclean spirit which years later affected my marriage bed. This was the reason sex had grown repulsive to me. What was done was unclean and unholy. The abortion had robbed us of the joyful and fulfilling sex life God intended for us to have. (Later on, the Lord dealt with me about how premarital sex had also given entrance to unclean spirits. I deal with this issue in a teaching God gave me on sex and intimacy.)

Making love with my husband was then better than any experience I ever had. It was clean, pure and holy. The only other time our sex life was affected by the abortion was some time before my "moment of truth" when the layer of violation was about to be exposed.

Many women who have had abortions struggle with sexual intimacy. Some say they feel dirty. Others feel violated and associate the sexual act with violation. Some fear getting pregnant and placing themselves once again in the position of having to abort. Others, like me, have no idea why sex is unappealing to them or why they are apathetic to it.

If you are a post-abortive married woman struggling to fully enjoy the sacred act of sex God ordained for you and your husband, I pray the Holy Spirit will use what I have shared here to reveal abortion's role, if any, in hindering mutual sexual fulfillment within your marriage.

Depression and Suicide

By far, the most debilitating consequence of the abortion I experienced was depression. While I recognize other factors unrelated to the abortion also contributed to my emotional lows, there is no doubt this relatively short medical procedure set me up for a myriad of ways to descend into the bowels of despair.

Thoughts of suicide filled my mind on many occasions. However, once I found out suicide was a sin, I resorted to putting myself in dangerous positions with the hope that somehow I'd inadvertently get killed. For instance, while in college, I began to wander the streets late at night hopeful some crazed criminal would sneak up on me and do the job. Tim, who was then my boyfriend, found about it after asking me where I had been. When I told him, he did something he rarely does: he got angry. He grabbed me by my arms and shook me, yelling, "What's the matter with you? Why would you do something like that?" I didn't know how to answer, so I just cried. He married me anyway. Go figure.

I have explained some of depression's effects on me earlier in the book and in this chapter, but here I will share the lowest low.

As we all know, pregnancy's effect on a woman's hormones can send her emotions traveling all across the globe - up, down and sideways. With my first three pregnancies, I suffered post-partum blues, but with my fourth pregnancy, I began sinking long before post-partum.

In the sixth month of the pregnancy, I developed guilt feelings about asking my husband for another child. Although he was content with two, my heart still longed for a large family. After my deliverance at the youth retreat, I had seen a picture in my mind of Tim and I with five children.

A friend of mine revealed a few years later she believed it was God's will for me to have five children. Shortly after this confirming insight, my daughter, Christen, who was about nine, surprised me by saying out of the blue, "Mom, there are supposed to be five kids in this family." Two other people had confirmed what I had envisioned, so I was pretty certain we should have five.

For some reason, though, during this fourth pregnancy, guilt for having asked Tim for another child badgered me constantly. He consented to having our fourth baby, but the nagging voice of condemnation offered its distorted rationale for his agreement: "He's just a nice guy and wants to make you happy." Then it would continue, "You, on the other hand, don't care about his happiness. He's struggling to make ends meet as it is, and now you've put more pressure on him. You know you're not the best mother and wife, and he has to bear much of the household responsibility; now he has to do even more. How could you do this to him? He'd be better off with someone else. You just create more hindrances to his success. He needs someone who will help him succeed." This torment continued day and night, driving me deeper and deeper into the "you're a bad wife and mother," and "you deserve to die" valley.

Obviously, even though I had thankfully been delivered from the hatred of children spirit, my mind had not yet been renewed about children.

Romans 12:2 says "And be not conformed to this world, but be ye transformed by the renewing your mind." (KJV)

There is a strong spirit of hatred of children in the world and it influences Christians and non-Christians alike. (I address this issue in a message

God gave me, which will take the form of a book in the near future.) The guilt about adding stress to my husband by asking for a fourth child is indicative of an unrenewed mind, conformed to this world and the satanically-inspired view of children. My baby was aborted because he was seen as a burden, a hindrance, and that message was subliminally imprinted in my own belief system.

In addition to dealing with this, the fear of losing my children and being unable to protect them went to a whole new level. The fear of losing the child in my womb in an accident or fire once he was born harassed me. I berated myself for adding another child to the three I already felt I couldn't protect. Feeling stupid and inadequate, I began to withdraw from friends and unbelievably, God.

The Lord is a God of hope, and I did not want hope. In times past, He would encourage me and tell me everything would be all right; but I would eventually end up doing something utterly stupid, disappointing myself, and Him too, or so I thought. I did not want encouragement. I did not want hope. I just wanted to give up. I wasn't worth the fight.

Having fully accepted this lie from the depths of hell, I allowed myself to drift away from Jesus. I wouldn't pray; and although my church attendance never waned, I tuned out the Word of God my pastor so accurately and anointedly preached. The Word could give me hope, but because I didn't want it, I wouldn't allow my heart to receive it.

To save on daycare costs, I stayed home with my three-year-old daughter during the day while my husband worked, and when he'd return home, I would work the 5 p.m. to 11 p.m. shift at my job. During the last few months of this pregnancy, it became almost impossible to drag myself out of bed before 11:00 a.m. Without any complaints, my husband prepared my two oldest children for school before he went to work, and my toddler-daughter quietly occupied herself with her favorite morning television shows, which unfortunately gave me the opportunity to stay in bed. I say it was unfortunate because it was during this time alone that feelings of inadequacy, worthlessness and depression hit me the hardest.

Every morning I'd lie there frustrated as I struggled but continually failed to devise a way to end my life without hurting my unborn child. There had to be a way . . . I just couldn't think of it. Then I'd consider how hurt my children would be if they lost their mother, and I'd recall how devastating the loss of my father was to me. I did not want to inflict that kind of pain on them.

Apprehension grew as I thought, *What if no one helped them through their grief? It would be awful if they internalized it and had to carry it alone.* (I thought these things not realizing this was exactly my problem - I had internalized not only my grief, but also my pain from the abortion and was suffering even then because of it.) Freely expressing themselves to adults was not easy for my children, so the idea of them suffering in silence was highly probable.

I couldn't do that to them. But then again, Tim would definitely marry again - surely a woman better suited for him - and his new wife's ability to be a wonderful mother would dispel my children's sense of loss and grief for their birth mother. Or would it? Maybe not.

Everyday, the same struggle. Everyday, the same frustration of being trapped - wanting to give up my miserable existence, yet not wanting to hurt my children, born and unborn. Because no means of accomplishing my goal materialized, I figured I could alleviate some of the pressure by leaving my husband and moving back to my mom's. This would give him the opportunity to find that "best-suited" wife he should have married in the beginning. He may hurt for a minute, but once he experienced his newfound freedom and a good wife, he would realize it was for the best. I figured he'd remarry within a year. Again, because I absolutely could not bear the thought of my children suffering due to abandonment by their mother - by death or otherwise - they, of course, would move with me. I may not have been the mother I had hoped to be, but I loved them and couldn't imagine life without them.

When I shared these plans with Tim, he let me know it was not for the best, and there was no way he was going to let me leave, especially with the kids. I'd bring it up again periodically, and he'd respond, "Would you stop saying that? We're not going to talk about that."

I had been slowly emotionally withdrawing from him, and he could tell I was despondent, so he'd ask me, "What's wrong?" I couldn't say much in response because it was too difficult to discuss. He wanted to help me, but didn't know how; and I wouldn't give any clues because I was not looking for help. Once I began talking about leaving, it was obvious it hurt him. It was horrible, but I was unable and unwilling to pull myself from the dreadful pit into which I seemed to be descending, and into which I was now dragging my family.

This new level of low continued until about nine months after my son was born. The emotional numbness had returned. I had a new baby I had to care for, and it looked like I wasn't going to leave, so I was back into "do what you have to do to function" mode. Long-abandoned painkillers, like alcohol, which the secret place I found in God had long ago dispelled, were trying to resurface. I envisioned myself buying a bottle of whiskey or wine and getting drunk out of my mind, although I never acted on it.

For over a year, not only I, but also my husband and children had been robbed of peace and the fullness of joy we should have experienced as a family.

As I mentioned before, I am aware the abortion's aftermath was not my sole escort to the depth of this low. Other emotional hurts played their respective roles, but the aftermath of the abortion was a major player. It contributed to my inability to see myself as a "good" mother. Good mothers don't kill their children or allow their children to be killed, at least not without a fight, right?

When ministering to post-abortive women, they will sometimes say to me, "But your abortion wasn't your decision. *I* made the decision to abort my baby(ies)." In essence, what they are saying is that I cannot relate to their feelings of guilt and their inability to forgive themselves because the decision to abort was not mine. This couldn't be further from the truth.

Although my mother was the primary decision-maker, I also made a decision. I decided to let it go. I have no idea what I could have done to change the decision. But in reality, what I could've, would've or should've done is of no consequence at all. The bottom line is that abortion - any abortion, regardless of whose decision - opens the door for guilt and condemnation to enter. This tormenting pair is included in the abortion package; they are inherent in the act. Depending on Satan's plot of destruction, they may begin their assault immediately, or they may wait, sometimes until thirty years down the road.

For me, they attacked and distorted my self-image as a mother. I was unable to identify them and the culprit that gave them entrance until the Holy Spirit exposed them; but they were there - guilt ever accusing me of being an unfit mother, and condemnation imposing a death sentence for my negligence.

One Sunday morning, the Lord spoke to me through my pastor while he preached. I was still pretty much there in body only, but the omnipotent and omnipresent God has a way of reaching us even when we think we are too far gone. In Psalms 139:7–10, David put it like this:

> *Whither shall I go from thy Spirit? Or whither shall I flee from thy presence? If I ascend up into heaven, thou are there: if I make my bed in hell, behold, thou art there. If I take the wings of the morning, and dwell in the uttermost parts of the sea; even there shall thy hand lead me, and they right hand shall hold me. (KJV)*

It doesn't matter how low you go. God, by His Spirit, will still lead and hold you. Even when I did not want to be found, He found me and spoke to me at my lowest low.

His words on this particular Sunday pierced through the armor of hopelessness surrounding my heart. He once and for all settled the issue that I am the wife He ordained for my husband. I am the one that will help him fulfill his destiny and purpose. I'm it. Therefore, I am the best-suited wife for him. Crying and halfway screaming, I made my way to the altar. The truth once again delivered me from the bondage in which lies had entangled me.

This glorious deliverance freed me from my depressed state, and I was ready to enjoy the brand new security in being the God-ordained help for my husband. However, I made a personal, inward resolution - I would never get pregnant again. I was done. I still believed it was God's will for me to have five children, and I still wanted five, but I could not risk sinking to the emotional low as with this last pregnancy and post-partum experience. If it happened again, I was certain I would die. There was no way I could endure it again. My dream had been stolen, and I had no desire to reclaim it.

The Rekindling

A little over a year after being delivered from the fear of losing my children, God thoroughly healed me through the experiences detailed in Chapters 1, and 5–8. This dramatic healing, however, did not enable me to recover my dream of having five children.

Four years after the post-abortion group ended and I began to walk in healing, my best friend called me on the phone and told me she dreamt about me. God normally speaks to her in dreams, so if she had a dream about me and felt impressed to tell me about it, I knew it must be significant. I listened intently as she proceeded to tell me she dreamt I had a baby.

A baby? No, she missed it this time. The food she ate before she fell asleep must have been speaking to her because there was no way I was having a baby. She said, "I don't know what it means, but I felt I needed to tell you I saw you with a baby."

Irritation churned within me. Why would God give her that dream, when He knew I let my dream of having another baby go? Then, I remembered something. A couple of weeks before, as I worked in one of the church's offices preparing the Sunday bulletin before morning worship, a four-year-old child approached me, patted my leg, looked up at me with angelic eyes and said, "Baby, baby, baby, baby." This particular child didn't talk much to anyone, and even today still doesn't, but for some reason he felt compelled to talk to me. Out of all the things he could have said, he just kept saying "Baby." I laughed it off then, but now it wasn't so funny. Someone else was saying "baby" to me.

"God, why are you doing this to me?" I asked now highly irritated. He knew it took a lot for me to settle for four children. "Why do you want to start this again? I was fine. Don't make me start thinking about this again." I made the decision not to listen, and I pushed the words of my friend and that child out of my mind.

The very next week, another sister with whom God also deals in dreams approached me after morning worship. She said, "I don't normally tell people about the dreams I have, but I feel God wants me to tell you what I dreamed about you. I dreamt you had a baby. I don't know if it represents a spiritual baby or a natural baby, but you definitely had a baby." I just stood there mute, staring at her. She and I were not close friends - we just spoke to one another briefly in church most times - and I knew she would not say something like this if she was not sure it had meaning.

Totally exasperated, tears welled up in my eyes, and I cried, "No, God. Please don't make me pick it back up again. I don't want to go through what I went through before. It was too hard. I don't want to be disappointed anymore."

For days I struggled. It was obvious He was speaking to me, but I was afraid. I always looked forward to being pregnant with high hopes of a pleasant pregnancy and post-partum, but I'd end up disappointed every time. With previous pregnancies, the voice of, "You're a terrible mother. Why would you have another child?" harassed me constantly, and it would go downhill from there. The last pregnancy almost killed me emotionally, and the prospect of that happening again struck terror in me because I knew I would not survive it.

While going through the post-abortion group, I suspected the severity of my depression during the last pregnancy was tied to the abortion. I knew beyond a shadow of a doubt, I had been healed, but what if the depression had been linked to something else? Could I risk it?

One evening while I sat in a church service, the Holy Spirit spoke to my heart and said, "The only thing keeping you from having another baby is fear. I have not given you the spirit of fear. Fear is not of me, and you cannot base whether or not you have another child on fear. It cannot be the determining factor. Don't you believe I can make everything all right? Trust me."

Of course He was right. I had let the enemy of fear block me from doing what I strongly felt in my heart God wanted me to do. My will broke, and I yielded. I closed my eyes, bowed my head and asked God's forgiveness. I also reaffirmed He indeed was Lord of my life, not fear, and I would trust Him to keep me whenever I was pregnant again.

After some months of waiting for my husband to catch the vision, I was pregnant. But not for long. I miscarried in the 11th week. Although disappointed and very sad, I noticed my grieving was not as severe as it had been when I miscarried 17 years before. Yes, I did grieve, and questioned God about why it happened, but I believe what I experienced was normal grief.

Four months later I was pregnant again. Quentin made his grand entrance, and at the age of 42, my dream of having five children was finally fulfilled. What a long, opposition-filled journey it had been!

The difference in my emotional state during and after my pregnancies before I was healed of the abortion's aftermath and this pregnancy was phenomenal. The lows and the post-partum blues never materialized. Five years after my healing, the final puzzle piece dropped in place; the final dot was connected. Much of the emotional suffering I experienced during and after pregnancy was related to the abortion.

The thief had been caught, and my precious possessions were being restored.

chapter 10

The Abundant Life

For twenty-two long years, I resided in the first part of John 10:10: "The thief comes but for to steal, and to kill and to destroy." (KJV) But Jesus changed my address. Now I happily dwell in the second part of that verse in which Jesus makes this astounding proclamation: "I am come that they might have life, and that they might have it more abundantly." Jesus came. Thank God, Jesus came. He came and boldly and lovingly entered the dark, smelly, secret place that housed my abortion's garbage. He removed the trash, and the life I now live I enjoy, not merely endure.

No longer am I abortion's slave, relegated to forever hauling its heavy baggage of shame, pain, loneliness, fear and grief. Jesus removed the burdens and healed the areas damaged by its weight.

Not only has He changed me, but He has miraculously transformed my oldest two children! Many days I cried and agonized over the inner pain I inflicted upon my children because of my fear, anger and self-perceived ineptness as a mother. I believed the injuries they sustained as a result of my bondage were irreparable. But God thought otherwise.

In Genesis 18:13–14 when Sarah laughed after being told she would bear a child in her old age, God said to Abraham,

> *Wherefore did Sarah laugh, saying, shall I of a surety bear a child, which am old? Is there any thing too hard for the Lord? (KJV)*

Is there anything too hard for Him? Is forgiving my sin of abortion and healing my wounded soul too hard? Is healing and restoring my children and our relationship too hard? The answer is an unequivocal, "No!" My entire family is experiencing healing and restoration, and if God did this for me, He certainly will do it for all.

As a matter of fact, I have witnessed God's faithfulness in transforming the lives of *every* post-abortive woman to whom I have ministered. I have come to understand that if a woman courageously emerges from abortion-induced isolation and shame to seek help, there is no way God will leave her hanging. He will reward her step of faith by touching her with His healing hand.

Abortion is not the unpardonable sin. Regardless of the circumstances surrounding your abortion - your choice, someone else's choice, one abortion, multiple abortions - one fact will forever ring true: God unconditionally loves post-abortive women. My life is a testament of His love, forgiveness, and mercy. Not only so, but I am evidence of His awesome power and willingness to heal and restore.

One of the most difficult challenges faced by post-abortive women in their healing journey is self-forgiveness. Many believe, "I don't deserve to be forgiven, and I can't (really, won't) forgive myself. I need to suffer because of my decision. I have to pay for what I did." This, however, is just another distortion the thief uses to rob us. While it is true that *none of us deserve* to be forgiven, please know that the unconditional love and endless mercy of the Father provided One to suffer and pay the price in our stead - namely, His only Son, Jesus. God, the Father, made an enormous sacrifice, and Jesus paid a high price for us. He was beaten to free us from our tendency to beat up on ourselves for past mistakes. He suffered shame, so we could approach the throne of God boldly and confidently. He endured the pain of crucifixion, so we could be healed. He poured out His life through His blood that was shed, paying the ultimate penalty for our sins, so we could live and not die. Do we then dare insinuate through our inability to forgive ourselves that His sacrifice was not enough? That the price He paid was insufficient to release us from our sin debt? God forbid. What a slap in the face that would be. The price has been *paid in full.* The work is complete. There is nothing else we can do to atone for our sins. His death has bought our life.

There is *life* after abortion - not a life condemned with shackles of guilt and shame, but abundant life. And this life is only found in Jesus. Only His blood can bring life to areas in us that have died. Only His precious blood can remove the stain of abortion. He alone is the Resurrection. Allow Him to come and bring you life.

I began this story describing God as a writer, producer and director, and as such, He knows the entire script, even how the story ends. While we may only see the scenes in which we are currently living, God has given us a promise in His Word which imparts hope for a favorable ending. Romans 8:28 puts it this way:

> *And we know that all things work together for good to them that love God, to them who are the called according to his purpose. (KJV)*

"All things" in this scripture means *all things.* If you love God and answer His call, He will work the good things and the bad things together for your good. Yes, even abortion.

For example, who would've thought that over two decades after having an abortion—something so ugly and selfish; something that many visibly and strongly endorse, yet when it's complete, imprisons women in a cell of hellish secrecy—who would've thought that after having done that, I would not only be admitting that I had one, but glorifying God because He is taking it, and turning it around to bring glory and honor to Himself.

As I lay on that table almost thirty years ago, experiencing what I thought was the absolute worst, God, who declares the end from the beginning, didn't just see the end of my child's life or the sin, but He saw down the road. He saw many years later; a day when His Lydia would stand up and unashamedly declare that God is merciful, that God is a healer, that God is a deliverer, and He can take your mistakes and turn them around for good. He saw the day when I would be sharing His mercy with other women through which they, too, would receive their healing. He saw my misery turned into ministry.

Who would've thought? I wouldn't have, but God did.

A Word to
Post-Abortive Women

As you read my story, certain emotions may have stirred in you: possibly guilt, unforgiveness, grief, a sense of loss, a sense of shame, regret, condemnation, or anger. If so, I encourage you to resist the urge to ignore or suppress it. Dealing with abortion's aftermath is difficult, I know; but the resulting healing and restoration are well worth it. Jesus awaits your call.

Please know that there are people who desire to minister to you and show the unconditional love of the Father. Below I have listed various organizations which can assist you further on your own healing journey.

Resources
Post-abortion healing:

Hearts at Rest
www.women-helping-women.net

The Abortion Recovery International Network
www.abortionrecoverydirectory.com

Rachel's Vineyard Retreats
1–877-HOPE-4-ME
www.rachelsvineyard.org

Healing Hearts Ministries
1–888–792–8282
www.healinghearts.org

Ramah International
www.ramahinternational.org

Deliverance:

An excellent array of books on deliverance is available on the online bookstore, *Arsenal Books.*
www.arsenalbooks.com

You may also contact me at:

Go Free Ministries
PO Box 972316
Ypsilanti, Michigan 48197
lydia@gofreeministries.com

Please visit my website at
www.gofreeministries.com

Contact Lydia Clarke at
lydia@gofreeministries.com
or order more copies of this book at

TATE PUBLISHING, LLC

127 East Trade Center Terrace
Mustang, Oklahoma 73064

(888) 361 - 9473

TATE PUBLISHING, LLC
www.tatepublishing.com